DISCOVER HEALTHY AGING AND LONGEVITY

HARNESSING EXERCISE, DIET, AND SELF-MOTIVATION FOR A LONGER, STRONGER, HEALTHIER LIFE

B. B. JOSEPH

CONTENTS

INTRODUCTION

The natural way of balancing life from the beginning to the end is aging; however, in this world where there are the sands of time that sweep youth and vitality along and leave behind the aftereffects of aging comes a remarkable phenomenon: *the Super Agers.*

These super-agers are quite exceptional individuals in this modern age. It is very remarkable whenever one comes across these individuals, who have been walking the earth for almost 8 to 10 decades. Picture it: an 89-year-old woman gardening while bending forward for over an hour with no signs of body aches or fatigue. Imagine a 90-year-old man moving briskly through the shopping aisles as he ticks off items on his list. It's almost as if there is a bounce in his step, along with the shine in his eyes and the smile on his face.

Can you imagine a life where we are free of the grip of aging and the symptoms and side effects are no longer a thorn in our side? Imagine going through old age without having to worry about sickness and declining cognitive and physical functioning. This is the journey we will take toward reaching these goals. *Discover Healthy Aging and Longevity* is a revolutionary guide written to aid you in discovering and walking the path that leads to an approach with evidence-based science, practical wisdom, and a transformative power you will realize within.

You may wonder: Why is this book anything different or exceptional? If this is a world where knowledge and information are lying around, you can get anything you need with just a few clicks on your smartphone, and bam! The internet is ready with a slew of answers and suggestions for you. You might think it's the same as every other book you are going to find on the market on healthy aging.

The short answer is: This is not the same as every other book out there. In fact, you can even go so far as to say that yes, even though it's much easier to read and understand, it is a far cry from a copy-and-paste from the internet.

Within these pages, you will find a treasure trove of well-defined and well-researched information, all geared toward assisting you toward healthier aging. It is unlike the conventional health tomes that are infamous for their medical jargon and robotic guidelines you're told to follow or implement in your lifestyle. This book is different due to the various disciplines, seamlessly merging science, psychology, nutrition, and fitness to create something almost similar to a work of art that will guide you toward healthy living with personalized steps to follow, all suited to your needs. You won't only be looking at scientific insights but also easy-to-follow guidelines, tangible strategies, and a treasure trove of resources that are all presented to you in an accessible manner. Look at this book as a companion that has all the tools you need to embark on this journey, not as the science textbook you read in 10th grade.

To be more thorough, within these pages, you will find the JOURNEY framework. This is an acronym that captures the essential steps you need to take to attain vibrant aging. Within these seven letters, you will discover a blueprint that unlocks the door to discovering the minute and larger details of how you can achieve improved mental and physical health, sound nutritional habits, increased motivation, an active lifestyle, and a renewed sense of control over the aging process.

The chapters within will follow this blueprint, and you will get to take away the step-by-step process of:

- Judging Aging—a chapter that invites you to challenge the traditional notions of growing older and embrace a new perspective on aging.

- Observing Your Health—a path that teaches you how to listen to your body's cues; identify warning signs, triggers, and deterioration; and take informed action.
- Unleashing Motivation—all about diving into the heart of this journey: motivation, the fuel that keeps burning that fire of hope within you to obtain lasting change.
- Revitalizing Through Exercise—a chapter that introduces a concept already known to you: how you can achieve vitality through a commitment to physical exercise.
- Nourishing Through Nutrition—another course similar to the one above that teaches you about the superheroes of the world: good food and nutrition.
- Enhancing Emotional Health and Social Interaction—where you dive into the connection between emotional well-being and aging.
- Yielding to Change—where you come to understand all the aspects involved and make peace with the knowledge as you incorporate it into your day-to-day living.

As your journey begins, you will be guided by the blueprint above, which serve as stepping stones for you to reach that life of vitality and purpose. Before you move on, though, keep in mind that this is not simply some guidebook. It's more of a compass that points in the proper direction. You will follow the needle, moving toward confidence, resilience, and an enriched sense of self. This is a promise of transformation and a path of life where aging is not a burden but a growing number. Aging is simply the next stage, another canvas on which you can paint the most vibrant picture you can.

If you have ever been plagued by the weight of vulnerability, the struggle of loved ones, and the desire to make your own path in this process known as aging, this is the right place. Here, you will find that catalyst for change, with a reservoir of well-thought-out and researched material all gathered for this one purpose: to help you rise above the limitations that old age might impose on you. All I ask is that you take the first step forward. Come with an open heart and a willing spirit as we reshape the way we have always approached aging. Let's create a new future—one brimming with vitality and well-being. This JOURNEY starts now.

1

JUDGING AGING

> *How old would you be if you didn't know how old you were?*
>
> — SATCHEL PAIGE

Let's imagine a scenario where you suddenly forgot your age and had to judge your mental, emotional, and physical aspects to guess what it was. How old would you be? Now, let's imagine another scenario: that this is not fiction but true. There are people out there whose age does not align with how they look, feel, or behave.

What if age was simply a number that had nothing to do with your physical and mental well-being? What if it had no relation to your body, stating when your bones, joints, and muscle mass should be deteriorating? What if age was a number that had no labels or strings attached? What if it came with no constraints every time it increased? This notion invites you to reconsider the narrative you have spun and believed about aging. This thought alone should encourage you to look beyond the changing calendar and ticking hands on the clock. You need to change your perspective as you dive into the tapestry of life and the journey of your later chapters.

In this chapter, we are going to explore the multifaceted nature of aging, the social perceptions that often color our understanding of aging, and the tangible potential to shape our lives toward healthier and more fruitful senior years.

WHAT DOES AGING MEAN?

To break it down, aging is all about going through a series of transformations. It is like a dance between the flow of time and our bodies' physical and emotional landscapes. It is a slow and gentle dance, almost mesmerizing. To put it simply, it is the biological canvas of the beginning right up until the last stages. It's an evolution from the development of a cell to genes and then an entire physical being. There is change and continuous growth until a stage when growth is inverse, and instead of getting stronger, there is a decline in overall well-being. Then again, aging does not only affect the physical. It isn't only the biological makeup of a human being. Aging also gets to lay her hands of slow deterioration on psychological and emotional aspects. Cognition, memory, and emotional resilience—all of these aspects are also affected with increasing age. Let's look into these changes in more detail (*Biological and Psychological Aspects of Aging*, n.d.).

Cognitive Function and Aging

As you age, it takes you much longer to process information and respond. Your memory skills decline as your ability to recall certain information in detail and with accuracy is affected. There is also diminished concentration; your focus can be cut short, and you become easily distracted and fatigued while keeping up. Eventually, there will be a decline in your executive functioning and language skills. Decision-making and problem-solving are affected. You will have difficulty finding the right word to use during conversation. It also becomes harder for you to understand complex words and phrases.

Psychological and Emotional State and Aging

Apart from the cognitive impact, the psychological and emotional aspects of your well-being are also affected by aging. You may experience irregular moods. It will become increasingly difficult to deal with and manage stress. There is a sense of loss and grief as you experience sadness at having lost a lot to time and aging. For example, your physique, your loved ones, your youth, etc.

Then again, not all impacts are negative. With age comes wisdom, maturity, and the ability to understand yourself better. You will be able to approach situations with more patience and insight compared to your younger self.

Biological State and Aging

When it comes to biology, every cell must age, and this can cause a variety of health issues or deterioration that can, either slightly or significantly, impact your lifestyle.

The first noticeable sign of aging is thinner, less elastic skin that is much more susceptible to wrinkle formation. Muscle mass decreases, and bone and joint health degrade. Posture is affected by the loss of strength in the spine, which makes the ligaments stretch and causes slouching.

Cardiovascular health is affected by thinner veins and more stress, which leads to high blood pressure and other heart-related conditions. Hormonal imbalances will begin to change the hormonal processing within your body. Men experience declining levels of testosterone, and women go through menopause with declining estrogen levels. The immune system is also impaired, becoming less efficient and slow. This makes you susceptible to developing infections, and it takes much longer to heal. Your sensory organs tend to undergo changes: Your vision blurs and hearing becomes a task. You gain weight easily as the metabolism slows. Decreasing muscle mass also leads to less energy usage. More calories tend to get converted into fat, which is then stored.

These changes are quite common, but it's important to keep in mind that each person is different. No two people experience the exact same changes or impact on their bodies. Yes, you could have similar side effects or symptoms, but no two people's experiences are exactly the same. The intensity and duration of symptoms may vary.

This can all sound rather disconcerting. After all, no one wants to age—or at least, no one wants to have a hard time facing old age and its companions. Living a life that is difficult and lacks the vibrancy of youth is depressing enough. However, this is not a life sentence. And it must be stressed going forward that growing old should not be a journey filled with prickly thorns and hidden pits. It does not have to be a chapter in your life when the only things to expect are health problems and mental conditions. It is true that life is going to gradually come to an end, but it does not stipulate in any history or biological textbook that a human being has to have a terrible aging journey.

In fact, we have all the tools and knowledge at our disposal, already waiting to be used, to ensure that the aging process is free of flare-ups that cause unwanted surprises. Each impact on your health or change in your physiology can be carefully monitored and addressed. You can add or change certain lifestyle habits to ensure that your life is moving toward healthy aging.

AMERICAN VIEWS ON AGING

Very often, the world looks at America, following her cues, almost like a symphony following a lead conductor. Yet, as the people follow, they also add their own unique harmony, enriching this global composition.

The same is true when it comes to views on aging. Over the past few decades, aging was mainly the cause of concern for women. They didn't want to show any signs of aging on their faces or their physiques, which started the explosion of the beauty industry, where there were cosmetics designed to cover signs of aging like wrinkles, patchy and dry skin, and so on. Then there was the evolution of fashion trends that made you lose the ability to tell just how old a woman was based on her fashion choices. The world evolved yet again with something new that flooded the market: various beauty products that went deep into the skin to help eradicate signs of aging. Despite all of this, there was one thing that stood the test of time, and that was self-care. Eventually, all women came to acknowledge the fact that they would only be able to stave off the side effects of aging by taking care of themselves, not just from outside but from within. After all, what we put in to our bodies reflects on the outside.

Currently in America, the views on aging have slightly altered for the opposite sex. In fact, when research was conducted, the statistics showed that recently, men have shown more interest in aging than women, but the reasons differ. For women, most are worried about aging due to their physical looks. For men, their worry when it comes to aging is declining health (Berger, 2017). The study went on to show that most youth these days tend to feel slightly negatively toward the aging population as well as the elderly, but older adults seem to have a positive feeling toward aging.

Other surveys were done relative to the elderly, and they found that over 60% of the older adult population went on to say that despite their age and physical appearance, they felt younger (*Growing Old in America: Expectations vs. Reality*, 2009). It was noted that the older they were, the younger they felt. On the other hand, most of the youth stated that they felt older than they actually were. Despite their opinions on what they felt, however, they did go on to investigate what different age groups considered to be the signs of old age. Those aged between their early 20s and early 40s voted on the fact that old age was proven by the inability to do certain tasks, the inability to live alone, and also by deteriorating health and well-being. A few did go on to state that getting old was related to having grandchildren, lacking control over their bowel movements, being retired, and having a lack of interest in sexual intercourse. The bottom line is that, based on these findings, many people tend to look at things individually. Some are scared of aging because of how it can affect their appearance and their health. Those who are nearing their late 40s are rather different in this regard, choosing optimism when considering their own aging process.

Society is almost like a mirror that reflects our own perspectives. In the US, those who have already started showing numerous signs of their aging process think differently. They appreciate and respect the elderly population and the aging process. So, yes, the perspective of every individual is different, and this is heavily influenced by their own age, background, and life experiences. Social media, which has long been associated with stigma and negativity, can also influence people's decisions and only recently has there been some light shed on the benefits of optimism and positivity when it comes to the natural aging process.

Regardless of society's opinions, it is not a universal truth. However, we should learn one thing: Our beliefs can both shape and be shaped by the world around us. For this reason, it is important that we understand the aging process and learn all we can about how the process works, what to expect, and how we can change the history of the process thus far. How do we rid ourselves of the fears that plague us as we see the sprinkling of gray hair and wrinkling skin?

CONFRONTING THE FEAR OF AGING

The fear of aging is an issue, and there is even a term for it —gerascophobia. For most people, it is an inevitable feeling. Aging is a journey we all embark on at some point in our lives. It has been a natural way of life since the very beginning. There is no way to avoid it or run away from it. It is something we all know is on the way—a road we must travel. And yet, this period does come with some fear and anxiety. This fear can weigh very heavily on your heart and mind. However, by looking at these fears straight on and unflinchingly, you get to transform them into sources of growth and empowerment. Otherwise, these fears would only lead to stress, anxiety, and depression (Dennis, 2021).

Common Fears Related to Aging

Declining Health

With age comes the deterioration of the physiological aspects of the body. This deterioration leads to numerous health issues, resulting in fear. Not knowing what to expect can leave you terribly uncomfortable and uneasy. The fear results from assumptions that you could possibly develop and experience chronic pain, physical limitations, and cognitive degradation. For example, an older person can worry about developing arthritis, diabetes, or any other heart condition due to old age. Should the person develop any, there will be a need to depend on loved ones, which can be very distressing once you start to think about it.

The impact that this will have on your mental well-being is fear, which leads to chronic stress and anxiety. You will also steadily become more aware of your bodily sensations, which cause worry as soon as you notice some kind of potential symptom. This will eventually result in an anxiety disorder, which makes it difficult for you to enjoy life or engage in any social activities.

Loss of Independence

Maintaining a healthy lifestyle is a crucial part of anyone's life. This is especially true when it comes to older people. It's only natural to fear the onset of a health condition when you know that it will cause you to no longer be able to care for yourself, both physically and mentally. Just imagine not being able to see to your needs, manage all of your daily activities, or even make decisions regarding your life. Aging in an unhealthy way tends to lead to various paths with various conditions and ailments popping up. This can be quite scary once you look at this way of life. Would anyone want to live this way? Would anyone want to lose their independence as their health takes it away from them?

The fear that comes from this loss of independence is mostly caused by the discomfort you feel whenever you imagine being in a position where you need to totally depend on another person, even for the simplest of tasks. The impact this has on your mental well-being is a strong push toward negative self-talk. You also begin to feel a sense of helplessness creep up on you as your self-worth diminishes. You may experience a loss of sense and purpose. This can lead to depression and anxiety symptoms worsening.

Picture an older person who is not able to drive because of deteriorating eyesight. Because of this, the person may begin to feel sad, frustrated, isolated, and dependent on others for various things: shopping, driving, handling money, and so on.

Loneliness

As we get older, it's only natural that our social circles begin to dwindle. We lose track of some of our friends, and with retirement, this issue tends to worsen. We become even more lonely. With physical limitations becoming more prevalent, there is very little opportunity to keep doing things when you can't meet up with other people. This leads to feelings of isolation and sadness.

The impact that this has on your mental well-being is chronic loneliness, which has been linked to an increased risk of developing depression and anxiety. We are social creatures, born to interact and speak to others frequently. Not being able to do this can contribute to a sense of hopelessness and have a negative impact on your cognitive functioning.

Try to imagine an older adult who lives on their own, has very limited social circles, and does not have the ability or motivation to participate in any activities that could lead to interaction with others. The person eventually begins to experience extreme feelings of emptiness and sadness. With prolonged exposure to these symptoms, the person could eventually develop clinical depression.

How to Address These Fears

From what you have seen thus far, these fears can lead to mental conditions. To maintain your emotional well-being, you must address these fears proactively.

- Have open discussions about the age-related fears you may experience with your family, friends, and members of your community. This way, you can garner the assistance and support you may need. Also, this will help others in this situation who do not know how to get the help they need.
- Seek professional help if you notice any kind of decline in your emotional health and well-being. Not only can they offer you solutions to the issue, but they can also provide you with some necessary guidance.
- Keep your mind in shape by engaging in a variety of physical and mental activities. This will promote an overall sense of well-being that can

counteract the negative effects of declining health, loneliness, and loss of independence.

- Build and enhance your social connections. If you already have friends and family who would like to see you, try to arrange a get-together. Try to join new groups or social organizations that will help you meet other like-minded people. You can even start your own club and get others to join you as you advertise what your group will be doing at your local community center.
- Work on your mind so it is resilient enough to empower you whenever you are facing age-related issues. You will be able to shift and move forward with a positive mindset and attitude.

The takeaway is that with aging comes the unexpected, but natural, onset of fear. There is a fear of diminishing health, loneliness, and lack of independence. We have already seen how aging can have profound effects on your mental well-being. Without addressing them appropriately, you will develop anxiety, depression, and chronic stress. All of this can contribute to the deterioration of your mental and physical health if it is not treated. As you move through this new chapter of your life, try to ensure that you have the right support strategies in place so you do not fall prey to the issues of aging. The only way to move forward from fear is to acknowledge it first. Only when you admit to something will you be able to fully face it and address it. You must ensure that this journey becomes a quest to face the fears head-on while transforming them into stepping stones toward healthy and happy aging instead.

THE IMPACT OF AGING ON HEALTH

The impact of aging goes deeper than the surface. It affects more than your appearance and your skin. Various aspects of your health are affected, but this is also largely influenced by several factors, which include your lifestyle choices, genetic factors, and your environment. It is true that your genes mostly play a role in determining how your body will age, but your lifestyle choices—such as the foods you eat, how much exercise you put into your daily routines, and what harmful habits you take part in or avoid—can also greatly contribute to how much your health stays constant, improves, or degrades. These impacts go deep, all the way down to the cellular and organ levels. Let's take a closer look at all of the symptoms that you can expect from the aging process (*Aging: What to Expect,* 2022).

Detailed Genetic, Environmental, and Lifestyle Factors

Genetics

Some individuals may be genetically predisposed to age-related health conditions. Others may have genes that offer some protection against certain conditions. With genetic factors, the body can alter or influence the rate of cellular aging, the efficiency of repair mechanisms, and the overall resilience of the body.

Lifestyle Choices

Your diet, physical activity, and consumption of alcohol and smoking, along with stress management strategies, play a vital role in the aging process. Poor lifestyle choices can speed up the aging process, decreasing the quality and longevity of life. Cells and organs age faster, which directly leads to chronic health conditions. On the other hand, active and healthy lifestyle choices help slow down the aging process. They promote better health in older years.

Environmental Factors

This includes a variety of situations and substances around you, like toxins, pollutants, radiation, etc., which can all cause and contribute to cellular degradation and aging. They directly impact aging. Then again, access to appropriate health facilities, social support networks, and financial stability can all aid in better living situations, which can decrease the aging process caused by certain harmful environmental aspects.

The Changes Within the Body

Cellular Changes

- Telomere shortening: The telomere is the protective cap at the end of your chromosomes. These caps tend to shorten each time a cell divides. This shortening is associated with cellular aging, which results in the cell's inability to divide and leads to tissue degeneration—the overall aging of all tissues in the body.
- Cellular senescence: Your cells are continuously dividing, and over time, changes result in a reduction in the replication rate. This directly affects tissue repair and regeneration, which increases the risk of developing age-related diseases. Telomere shortening is another cause of this senescence. Both of these issues cause inflammation, tissue dysfunction, and the progression of any other age-related conditions.
- Oxidative stress: This is where the accumulation of oxidative damage from free radicals leads to cellular dysfunction and damage to cellular components. This includes your DNA, lipids, proteins, and more. This stress is also known to be implicated in various age-related diseases by promoting DNA mutations, disrupting lipid membranes, and eventually accelerating cellular aging.

Organ-Related Changes

- Your musculoskeletal system declines. The gradual loss of muscle mass, sarcopenia, contributes to muscle weakness, decreased mobility, and an increased risk of falling. This occurs because of the decrease in the number and size of muscle fibers and the reduction in muscle protein synthesis.
- With aging, your bone density also decreases. There is an imbalance between bone resorption, or breaking down, and bone formation. This results in osteoporosis, where the internal structure is weaker and more susceptible to fractures.
- Your arteries become less flexible and more rigid with age. This can cause high blood pressure as the blood flow decreases. There is also a decreased level of pumping that is caused by old age changing the structure and functioning of the heart.
- Your lung function declines, and there is a reduced ability for the lungs to exchange gases efficiently. This is one of the main reasons why older adults tend to develop respiratory infections.
- Neurons in your brain also undergo degradation. This leads to declining memory and cognitive function. Neuron degredation can also lead to

neurodegenerative diseases like Alzheimer's and Parkinson's.

- The immune system and endocrine system are also affected. The decrease in the function of immune cells decreases their ability to fight against disease. With age come hormonal changes, which can cause drastic changes and impact the normal functioning of the body. Certain processes will be affected, like the usage and digestion of glucose, sugar, and erythritol, which can result in abdominal weight gain and lead to heart health conditions.

The effects on the organs and cells of the body are a multifaceted process. It is driven by varying molecular and physiological changes. Now that you understand how environmental, lifestyle, and genetic conditions can affect your body during the aging process, you can come up with strategies to ensure that you do not have a difficult aging process.

INFLAMMATION, CHRONIC ILLNESS, AND PAIN IN AGING

When it comes to aging, you will most likely have to experience at least one of the following: inflammation, pain, or some kind of chronic illness. Some people are lucky enough to have no issues, but they are the rare ones.

The main issue is that we either do not take care of our bodies throughout our lives and the aftereffects show in our older years, or the genetic issues that are unavoidable take precedence. There are ways to combat these situations, but before we look into them in detail, it's time to delve into this chapter of the aging process to understand just why it happens.

Inflammation and Chronic Illness

Some people experience something called inflammaging. This is where your body naturally becomes inflamed, and the inflammation is more prevalent and sustained. This is supposed to be one of the main causes of chronic illness (Ferrucci & Fabbri, 2018).

The onset and ongoing effects of inflammation cause tissue damage, impaired organ functions, cardiovascular disease, diabetes, arthritis, and neurodegenerative diseases.

Cellular Senescence and Inflammation

We have already looked at this issue and how it leads to inflammation. These cellular senescent cells release inflammatory molecules known as cytokines, which create a pre-inflammatory environment. Cytokines are responsible for damaging surrounding cells and tissues. This all eventually leads to the progression of chronic illnesses (Zhang & An, 2007).

Chronic Illness and Pain

It's more common for older adults to develop chronic illnesses since inflammation often causes a variety of conditions, like diabetes, hypertension, heart disease, arthritis, and chronic obstructive pulmonary disease (COPD). These issues and their related symptoms cause ongoing health conditions and challenges. There will be a frequent need for quality and quick medical care. There is also the reduced quality of life that is inevitable and associated with various conditions.

Pain

Chronic illness can come with one very terrible side effect: persistent and ongoing pain. There are other conditions that can also limit your mobility and cause significant discomfort. These are conditions like arthritis, back pain, and neuropathy. Pain is not only going to affect your physical well-being; it also has psychological and emotional implications. It could lead to anxiety and depression. There is also a decreased ability to engage in daily activities.

The Impact on the Quality of Life

With pain and chronic conditions come quite a few impacts on life and its quality as well. Let's look into these in more detail.

- With chronic illness and pain, there is a decline in the functioning of your body. It makes it difficult for you to perform tasks and daily activities. You may no longer be capable of living independently as it becomes increasingly difficult to take care of yourself. These mobility issues and fatigue, coupled with pain, can make it difficult for you to exercise, move, and engage in social activities.
- Continuously bearing and having to deal with psychological issues and pain can start wearing down your psychological well-being. This will accompany the discomfort that makes life uncomfortable. Living like this will cause feelings of frustration, helplessness, and depression. You may also experience anxiety when it comes to the constant need to find ways to manage your symptoms and conditions.
- The combination of chronic conditions, pain, and mobility issues can often result in social isolation. You will begin to withdraw from social activities because you may want to avoid the challenges posed by any conditions you may have. This will lead to even more health concerns arising from feelings of loneliness, like emotional distress.
- With chronic illnesses coming about more frequently and persistently, you will require urgent or frequent medical treatment, appointments, and facilities. This will become an emotional, physical, and financial burden. There

> will be a heavy strain placed on you as the need to depend on the medical world becomes more pressing.

There is an interplay between inflammation, chronic illnesses, and pain. This is one of the most difficult aspects to accommodate because of the natural issues that come along with aging. To address these challenges, you will need to come up with a comprehensive approach that includes medical management, pain management strategies, lifestyle modifications, and social support to avoid the progression of certain chronic diseases, pain, inflammation, and a decline in mobility and quality of life. We will look into these aspects in detail in the following chapters.

HOW CAN WE DELAY THE ONSET OF CHRONIC DISEASE?

Despite all of the darkness and negativity that engulfs you when you begin to journey into old age, there is a beacon of light that can help bring you out of the darkness and onto the positive side. Remember, the onset of chronic diseases does not have to be irreversible. It is more like an opportunity for choice. Always keep in mind that your lifestyle choices and decisions are what lead you down the path of healthy aging or life's deteriorating quality in old age.

Delaying the Onset of Chronic Diseases Through Healthy Lifestyle Choices

Aging is a natural process. Certain changes will occur within your body that you just can't control. However, there is a way to slow or delay the process of some, and there is also a way to prevent certain impacts on your health from coming to pass. This can be done by changing some of our lifestyle habits. You can improve the quality of your life, and all you need to do is develop some new habits or change or eradicate some old ones completely (Elwood et al., 2013).

- Change your diet to include more fruits, vegetables, whole grains, lean proteins, and healthy fats. These nutrient-dense foods provide you with essential benefits. For example, maintaining a healthy weight, reducing inflammation, and supporting positive immune function and health.
- Regular exercise is also very beneficial. It prevents chronic disease by maintaining a healthy body weight, strengthening bones and muscles, improving cardiovascular health, and supporting cognitive function.
- Smoking and drinking alcohol can cause quite a few health conditions. They even lead to chronic diseases, weakened immune systems, and inflammation, all of which can eventually result in

a horrible loss of health or even death. Avoiding harmful habits can improve longevity and quality of life.

- Stress is often termed "the silent killer." Many people are aware of this, but even so, they do not know when they are overstressed or do not make any effort to reduce their stress levels. Engaging in relaxation techniques can be quite beneficial when it comes to the healing process. You can practice meditation and deep breathing exercises to help calm your mind and slow the effects of aging. They always have some kind of positive impact on your overall health.
- Getting enough sleep is another habit we need to incorporate into our daily lives. Less sleep equals decreased health, cognitive function, and emotional well-being.
- Getting regularly checked and screened is a great way to identify any risk factors and prevent developing any major conditions. This way, you and your doctors can stay up to date on your health and ensure that you are following a healthy diet and physical health habits and that you are on the right path for your health journey.
- By maintaining strong social connections and staying connected with friends, family, or community members, your mental and emotional well-being is promoted. This reduces the risk of certain emotional well-being-related conditions

as you eliminate isolation and loneliness from your life.

- By keeping up with the preventive healthcare system, you can avoid developing certain health conditions. For example, by getting the recommended vaccinations and getting timely screenings done, you can eliminate the risk of developing pneumonia, influenza, and even certain types of cancer.

By adopting all of these lifestyle habits, you can positively influence your health outcomes as you age. You not only delay the onset of chronic health conditions, but you also improve your body's resilience, improve your overall quality of life, and promote more positive aging experiences. This will all help lead to a more fulfilling and healthier life in your later years.

The effects of aging are vast and nuanced. They are painted with colors that span from vibrancy to vulnerability. In the next chapters, we are going to delve even deeper into the aging process, looking into unearthing the keys that lead to restoring a sense of vitality. As we move on, it's time to equip ourselves with the knowledge of how we can observe our health with clarity and the tools to maintain our own healthy lifestyle.

2

OBSERVING YOUR HEALTH

> *Our bodies are our gardens, and our wills are our gardeners.*
>
> — WILLIAM SHAKESPEARE

Try to imagine yourself as a gardener, but instead of tending to plants, you are nurturing the incredible and unique garden that is your body. Just as for every skilled gardener, you need to have some knowledge and resources to understand and offer your mind some sprinkling of enthusiasm to ensure that you know what you are doing and that you are keeping your garden healthy and well, serving its every need. Only you have the power to tend to this garden; it is your sole responsibility.

In this chapter, we are going to dig deep into the magical world of your body's garden and make it thrive.

GET TO KNOW YOUR BODY'S BUILDING BLOCKS

This section serves more like a backstage pass that gives you VIP access to understanding your body and what makes it move: your muscles, bones, and ligaments. These three parts are the rock stars of your physical health, especially since they all have tales to tell.

Muscle, Bones, and Ligaments

Your muscles can be thought of as the stewards of your body. They are always ready to spring into action. The bones are the scaffolding that keeps you upright, and the ligaments are the trusted connectors that hold it all together. However, there is a twist. These parts all get some kind of makeover as you age. Let's explore these changes and how they can impact your life. Let's also look at the ways you could use them to keep them in fit and functioning shape.

Muscles

Muscles work like the engines of the body. They contract and relax to help you move. Every movement you are capable of—walking, jumping, twitching—requires the movement and activity of a muscle.

Bones

You could picture your bones as the sturdy frame that keeps the body up and protects the vital organs within.

Your bones provide structure and help store and create essential vitamins and nutrient cells, like the red blood cells that are formed in the bone marrow and are essential for absorbing oxygen from the lungs, moving it throughout the body, and returning deoxygenated blood to the lungs to repeat the process.

Ligaments

This part of the body is similar to glue. The role of ligaments is to link the muscles, joints, and bones together.

The issue here, though, is that as you age, every part naturally begins to degrade. So, the best way to manage any situation that either flares up or starts as a slight problem is to observe or pay attention to it. Muscles lose their mass, bones lose density, and ligaments need some TLC as their stretchiness and tautness become impaired.

From these issues come challenges. Your strength and posture deteriorate. You will no longer be able to move easily, and your flexibility will also become nonexistent. Your body will start to hunch over, causing the organs in your body to squash against one another. Your quality of life will decrease gradually, and you will no longer be able to maintain an independent and vibrant lifestyle. You will need help doing day-to-day tasks, as there will be no way for you to easily move your arms or stand up.

With the proper care, however, you will not face as many challenges.

MEASURING YOUR FITNESS

Now it's time to move on to your personal fitness playground. You get to complete some fun tests to see how well your body is performing. This also helps you measure your fitness levels—how strong, flexible, and able you are. It doesn't have to be a chore, but more of an adventure, with the prize being a healthier, more vibrant you!

The Tests

Test 1: Push-Up Test

This is done to measure your upper-body strength. You should count how many push-ups you can do in one go.

- Begin by warming up to prepare your muscles. You can do some light stretches, such as marching on the spot, light walking, jumping jacks, or jogging for at least three to five minutes.
- Get your body in the proper position. Your hands should be placed slightly wider than shoulder-width apart. Keep your body straight, aligned from your head and back down to your legs. This position will help keep your core engaged. As you get ready to perform the test, remember to practice belly breathing (deep breathing, inhaling

through your nose, and exhaling through your mouth).

- You will execute the test by leaning your body toward the ground with your elbows.
- Keep your back straight as you do the movements, lowering yourself until your chest nearly touches the floor.
- Push your body back with your arms fully extended.
- Perform as many of the movements as you can in proper form (your back should be straight and not arching).
- Your aim should be to do as many push-ups as you can until you can no longer do them properly. You can also do them as many times as you want until you reach a predetermined number.
- Try to keep track of how many push-ups you've completed with good form. This should be an indicator of your upper-body strength.

Test 2: Balance Test

This test is done to gauge your balance and assess your stability.

- Find a quiet place with an open space and a stable surface.
- Remove any obstacles or hazards from the area.

- Stand up straight with your feet close together and your arms hanging loosely by your sides.
- Lift one foot off the ground, bending your knee at a 90-degree angle.
- Keep your body balanced on one leg while keeping your arms at your sides or on your hips.
- You can close your eyes if you prefer, but make sure that if you lose your balance, you will not bump into anything dangerous.
- As you keep balanced on one leg, try to keep track of how long you can maintain your balance. Use a timer to help you keep track of the seconds that tick by.
- Once done, you will need to perform the same test on the other leg. As you keep track of how long you can maintain your balance, you will gain some insight into your overall balance.

Test 3: Flexibility Test

Flexibility tests are done to measure how limber you are.

- Begin by finding a quiet and open space with a comfortable surface for you to sit on. This can be a yoga mat or a carpet.
- Reach forward as you try to touch your toes without bending your knees.

- Go as far as you can without hurting yourself or pulling your muscles uncomfortably. If you cannot reach your toes, this is fine.
- You will need to record the distance between your fingertip and your toes. This is an indicator of your hamstring flexibility.
- You can repeat these stretches on other muscle groups to see how far you can go. Try your shoulders, back, and quadriceps.
- With each stretch, you gain insight into your overall flexibility.

These tests will provide you with valuable information about your physical fitness levels. They can also serve as a baseline against which you can track your progress over time. As you try out these tests and get on to the exercises later on, you must remember to prioritize your safety and ensure that you're doing the exercises with the proper form. You could also consult with a fitness professional if you feel uncomfortable about doing these tests because of any physical limitations.

Keep in mind that these tests are like little adventures on this journey that you can do within the comfort of your own home. They're there to help you evaluate your physical and mental levels as you set goals to improve yourself.

NURTURING YOUR RESPIRATORY HEALTH

This is the second part of the journey when it comes to understanding your health. Here, we are going to delve deep into the details of your respiratory health—the breath of life itself.

As we age, all parts of our body will begin to deteriorate, including our lungs. With proper care and maintenance, your health and lungs can avoid the chronic issues related to aging. Let's explore the why and the how.

The Marvel of Your Lungs

Your lungs are essentially known for their ability to exchange air, and they work tirelessly to ensure that your body receives the oxygen it needs to survive. These organs can be compared to fine wine—as they age, they become more delicate. For this reason, it's vital that you understand how they weaken and what complications may arise as you age. The issues that you can face include:

Reduced Lung Capacity

If you had to use a visual example, picture your lungs as balloons. They inflate and decrease in size as air goes in and out. Over time, with use, the balloon does not inflate as fully as it used to, nor does it have the ability to keep its shape for too long. This will affect your ability to hold your breath, and it will also affect your ability to breathe deeply. To combat this, you can do some simple exercises, like deep breathing, to help maintain your lung capacity.

Asthma

Some people can develop asthma later in life. This could be for varying reasons, for example:

- exposure to allergens, pollen, and other irritants or any new environmental factors at home or work
- respiratory infections like viral infections or pneumonia, which can lead to inflammation and hypersensitivity of the airways
- new or worsening allergies that cause inflammation and constriction of the airways
- toxic changes in lifestyles like breathing second-hand smoke from cigarettes and smoking

To combat these issues, you would need to visit your healthcare provider and obtain the prescribed medication that will help alleviate the symptoms you are experiencing. You should also work hand in hand with your doctor to determine what your triggers are. Avoiding them can help reduce the exacerbation of your symptoms. You should also strive to make positive lifestyle changes that will support your lung health. Track or monitor your symptoms in a journal and try to learn how to use your inhaler correctly. You must stay up to date on vaccines and other preventive methods that can help manage your symptoms.

Asthma is properly managed by using a holistic approach. With the help of your doctor, using your medical history, adjusting lifestyle habits, and finding out what your triggers are, you can come up with an approach that will help manage the condition effectively, allowing you to live an active and healthy life.

Lung Infections

With age, your body's ability to fight against diseases is also drastically affected. A lack of movement, living a sedentary lifestyle involving unhealthy diets, and not putting in any effort and allowing our bodies to just wither away, reduce our body's ability to fight off almost any kind of viral or bacterial attack. Some of the reasons why we develop infections and are more susceptible to them include:

- As we age, our weakening immune system does not respond in the same way it did in our younger years.
- Chronic health conditions weaken the respiratory system and cause inflammation. This makes the lungs even more vulnerable to infection.
- As a side effect of aging, declining lung function causes declining elasticity and respiratory muscle strength, causing the lungs to clear mucus

inefficiently and also hindering their defense against infections.

- With reduced mobility and a lack of exercise, which are very common in aging adults, there is a high increase in the risk of developing pneumonia or a lung infection.

To combat these issues, you should:

- Make sure that your body has all the up-to-date vaccinations. This is especially true for the flu and pneumococcal vaccines.
- Practice good hand hygiene. With the recent pandemic, we saw just how important cleanliness can be in the fight against disease. We never know what type of virus or bacteria our hands will come across during our daily adventures. Washing your hands and ensuring that they are clean can help prevent a wide array of lung and other infections.
- Keep updated on information surrounding flu and pneumonia and take the necessary precautions, like getting your vaccines, ensuring that you are properly dressed, and keeping your body well nourished and active to fight off any disease.
- Try to avoid or quit smoking so your children can maintain their health and safety. Always keep in mind that another significant effect of smoking is that it speeds up the aging process in your internal organs. Cigarettes also contain harmful chemicals

known as carcinogens. These toxic substances can cause dormant cancer cells to awaken and spread the disease.
- Maintain a healthy and well-balanced diet and lifestyle. With the required amount of hydration and the management of symptoms and conditions with the prescribed medication, you will be on your way to healthy aging.

Now that you know more about how aging can lead to lung degradation and other health-related issues, it's time to move on to assessment testing to measure the health levels of your lungs.

ASSESSMENT TESTS FOR RESPIRATORY HEALTH

Knowing how healthy your lungs and their functioning are helps you take note of your current health state and then move on from there, knowing exactly what you need to do to change the direction from negative to positive. Let's get started.

Lung Function Tests

Spirometry is a test that measures your lung capacity and airflow. To begin, the doctor or technician will ask you to take a deep breath in and then exhale as hard as you can. This is done using a tube that you put your mouth around, and the measurements are all recorded on the machine the tube is connected to. The machine will record how much air you can take in and how much you exhale, as well as how quickly.

Breathing Diagnostic Tests

Bronchodilator response testing is a test that measures how well your airways respond to medication. First, you will need to do a spirometry test and then inhale bronchodilator medication. Once this is done, after a specific period of time, you will need to undergo a spirometry test again. This will help monitor whether your lungs can improve their function with medication. This can help prevent conditions associated with your lung health, like asthma.

Peak flow measurement is a type of test that helps track how fast you can exhale air. First, you will need to stand upright and take a deep breath. You will then need to seal your lips around a mouthpiece and then blow out as hard and fast as you can. This will be done a few times to generate an average score.

These are some of the tests that you could do to get insight into your respiratory health. With this knowledge, you walk forward and are one step closer to maintaining your lung health. You'll be ensuring that your breath is healthy and that you age without the natural decline in respiratory health, as you are already skilled in how to combat any issues.

CIRCULATORY HEALTH

It's time to explore the fascinating world of the circulatory system. If you had to imagine the way it worked, try to picture it as a bustling highway of life. The heart is at the center, pumping blood to every part of your body. The whole circulatory system is well circulated. The flow of the blood through the veins and arteries—all aspects working together in harmony to ensure that you are alive and that every part of the body, internally, gets what it needs. Essential nutrients move to where they are needed and waste is excreted. Every process in the body is possible because of the circulatory system.

As we age, even this beautiful system is affected. Your heart has to work harder to do its job. Blood vessels lose their elasticity, and the whole system is affected in some way or another.

Unlocking Medical Terms

Let's look at the medical side of things to see how age affects the circulatory system, the names of the leading causes, and what these issues are known as so you better understand this side of your health and well-being.

Cholesterol

This is a very common term, and if you haven't heard about it in your high school biology class, then you most likely heard about it in an advertisement about heart health or at your local doctor's office. Cholesterol is necessary when it comes to building cell membranes, producing hormones, and forming bile acids to help digest food. However, like every other aspect of the body, the levels must be stable to ensure that your body is functioning in perfect order.

As you age, cholesterol levels can be affected. Your body is unable to regulate your levels, and high levels of LDL or low-density lipoprotein (bad cholesterol), can affect your circulatory health. Bad cholesterol affects your arteries and can clog your blood vessels. This is known as atherosclerosis and leads to stiffened arteries. It increases the risk of developing heart disease over time, and other organs are also affected, as there is a decrease in the amount of oxygen they receive.

To ensure that your health is at its optimum level, especially your cholesterol levels, you will need to closely monitor them through blood testing.

Blood Sugar Levels

This is also more commonly known as your blood glucose levels. Glucose is what we get from eating carbs and sugar, and it is transformed into energy in the body. When we are active, our energy is used up. However, when we don't use it up, it is transformed into fat and stored. Maintaining the right levels of glucose in your body is important for your overall health; after all, every part of your body needs energy to function properly.

As we age, it is difficult to maintain blood sugar levels. There is a higher risk of developing certain conditions, like prediabetes or type 2 diabetes. High levels of blood sugar can cause a variety of health issues, like poor vision, kidney issues, and heart disease. Age and the habits caused by an aging body, such as a lack of exercise and poor diet choices, can affect how your body regulates glucose. For this reason, it is imperative that you monitor your blood sugar levels and ensure that they are kept in check.

Blood Pressure Levels

Blood pressure revolves around your cardiovascular health. To put it simply, it is the force of your blood pumping as it pushes against the walls of your arteries and your heart continuously pumps it to and through your entire body.

With an appropriate blood pressure level, everything flows smoothly. As you age, however, the natural beat of your heart, the flow of blood, and the pressure of the blood can be affected. In some cases, it is a minor change, but for others, it can be quite drastic and debilitating. Your blood vessels stiffen, which will lead to hypertension or high blood pressure. When this happens, the beat and force of your heart have to increase so the blood is able to get past these narrow spaces. It becomes too fast and forceful, eventually putting a strain on your circulatory system.

Many are unaware of just how damaging high blood pressure can be, as it severely impacts the delicate lining of your arteries and makes them more susceptible to plaque buildup and narrowing. Hypertension will eventually lead to an increased risk of developing heart disease, stroke, and other circulatory problems. You could imagine it as though it's a drum beat that is becoming more erratic and overpowering as it disrupts the harmony of your body's ensemble.

For these very important reasons, as you age, you should maintain a harmonious balance of blood pressure. You should monitor your levels, as well as maintain healthy lifestyle habits, which include a healthy diet, regular exercise, stress management, and a holistic, healthy approach to life. All of this will help keep your heart beating steady and your circulatory system in harmony.

Assessment Tests for Circulatory Health

When it comes to maintaining circulatory health, knowledge is the most potent instrument. Let's look at the tests and assessments you can use to monitor the rhythm of your heart and vascular health.

- Cholesterol screening is a test performed to assess your cholesterol levels so you and your healthcare provider can come together and make informed decisions about your diet, medication, and lifestyle. We have also looked at this previously but as we age, higher levels of bad cholesterol are noticed and are associated with heart disease. Aging also affects the good cholesterol levels in your body and by managing these levels, you will be able to prevent any age-related cardiovascular issues.
- Blood sugar tests help you understand and manage your glucose levels more effectively. Note that with high levels of glucose in your system, almost every organ in your body is put in harm's way. As we age, there is a higher risk of developing type 2 diabetes. Aging can also lead to increased insulin sensitivity and decreased metabolism, which cause weight gain. High blood sugar levels can also lead to serious complications like heart disease, kidney disease, and nerve damage. For all of these reasons, it's important that regular blood sugar testing, such as fasting blood glucose and hemoglobin A1C tests, be performed regularly.
- Blood pressure monitoring is the most basic and common system used to keep an eye on your heart rhythm. The main reason why these tests should be done regularly is because certain changes affect

the blood vessels, as we have already seen how plaque buildup increases. Hypertension is a major risk factor for cardiovascular disease. By monitoring your blood pressure levels, you can detect certain conditions early on and either maintain or eliminate them.

MENTAL HEALTH ASSESSMENT

As we grow older, another major part of our body is at risk of deterioration. Our mental health is just as vital as any other part of the body. Now it's time for us to discuss the importance of assessing your emotional strength and stress levels, as their rising and conflicting levels can only lead to mental health deterioration and related conditions.

Why It Matters

Try to imagine your mental health as the conductor of your life's orchestra. It is the conductor that gives the direction of the flow of fully functioning processing, joy, and fulfillment. When your mental health is affected, certain functions and processes are hindered. Your body ceases to exist the same way it did in your younger years. Your body is no longer able to move as easily. It takes much longer for you to digest your food. It is much more difficult for you to think of things that are usually common knowledge... This is just the gist of it. When it is affected, tremendous changes in your physical and mental health can and will happen, not to mention the increased risk of developing conditions like Alzheimer's, dementia, schizophrenia, and more.

To ensure that your mental health is still in good shape, you must keep an eye on your stress levels. Stress is the instrument that is used to break down peace and tranquility within your body. It affects not only your thinking patterns but also the rhythm of your everyday existence.

It's not that stress is some alien concept that is going to single you out and affect your mental health. It is more of a natural response that every human being has when experiencing challenging situations. Stress every once in a while can be considered natural, but chronic stress is the problem. This type of stress has detrimental effects on your physical and mental well-being. Recognizing the signs and then employing effective stress management techniques are very important when it comes to maintaining a balanced and healthy lifestyle. Some of the most common signs of stress include (*Signs and Symptoms of Stress*, 2022):

- muscle tension
- pain
- headaches
- migraines
- fatigue
- trouble sleeping

- digestive problems
- increased blood pressure and heart rate
- irritability
- mood swings
- anxiety
- nervousness
- racing thoughts
- constant worry about the future
- lack of concentration
- memory issues
- overeating or undereating
- increased use of alcohol or smoking
- decreased productivity
- restlessness
- isolation

To manage stress, you can try several types of techniques to mitigate its effects. These include:

- Deep breathing and relaxation techniques help calm your nervous system. Progressive muscle relaxation, which is a side effect, will also help reduce your muscle tension.
- Exercising regularly is very beneficial, as physical activity helps your body release endorphins. This is a natural stress reliever. You can try to incorporate activities like yoga, meditation, and other exercise routines you enjoy.

- Maintaining a healthy lifestyle is very important. Some habits to develop include eating a balanced diet, staying hydrated, limiting caffeine and alcohol consumption, and ensuring that you get enough sleep.
- Ensuring that your time management is prioritized and dealt with efficiently makes it much easier for you to avoid stressful situations. To prioritize this, complete important tasks and create a schedule to avoid feeling overwhelmed. You could also break it down into smaller, more manageable steps.
- Seeking social support by talking to friends, family, or even a therapist, can help decrease your stress, as well as provide you with emotional support. Practicing mindfulness techniques and meditation helps you stay mentally focused in the present and reduces anxiety. These practices also help promote relaxation and mental clarity. By setting realistic goals for yourself, you can decrease stress because they are achievable.
- You should always celebrate each and every achievement, no matter how small.
- Should your stress become overwhelming, it's important that you consider seeking help from a professional, which includes a counselor or therapist.

Assessment Tools for Mental Health

As is the situation with most of your well-being, obtaining knowledge empowers you to take control of your health. The same is true when it comes to your mental health. Here are some of the assessment tests and tools that are used:

- General mental health screening is a diagnostic tool that is used to evaluate your overall mental health.
- Stress assessment is used to identify stresses in your life, as well as learn how to manage them effectively.
- Depression and anxiety screenings are used to detect symptoms of depression and anxiety, help you seek guidance, and find the right methods of managing these conditions.

UNDERSTANDING AND ASSESSING YOUR MICROBIOME

Many are unaware that a specific ecosystem that is bustling with inhabitants lives within their bodies: the digestive system. Let's look at it in detail (*The Microbiome,* 2017).

Over the years, scientists have unveiled a fascinating world known as the microbiome. This is a very complex ecosystem with trillions of microorganisms: bacteria, fungi, and other microbes that all reside within our bodies. The system primarily exists in the gastrointestinal tract, skin, and various mucosal surfaces. The system can be referred to as a hidden universe that plays a pivotal role in managing and maintaining our overall well-being.

These trillions of microorganisms coexist within the body. It's not just a collection of foreign invaders but an important part of our bodies. It is not seen as separate; it's something that exists within you and functions as an organ within your body. It assists with various important functions, such as aiding in digestion, boosting the immune system, synthesizing vitamins, and even influencing your mood and behavior.

So why is it important?

- A balanced gut microbiome is very important when it comes to digestion and absorption of nutrients.
- The microbiome is responsible for breaking down complex carbohydrates, producing enzymes, and maintaining your gut health.
- The microbiome also acts as a barrier against harmful pathogens, as it helps train the immune system to respond appropriately.
- An imbalance in your microbiome can lead to increased susceptibility to infections and autoimmune diseases.

- The microbiome also plays a role in your metabolism, as well as weight regulation. Without it, you will quickly fall into obesity and develop metabolism disorders. This is especially true if you aren't constantly aware of your diet and what it consists of.
- The microbiome also helps to prevent the colonization of harmful bacteria. This reduces the risk of diseases like irritable bowel syndrome, Crohn's disease, and colorectal cancer.
- The gut-brain connection, which is also known as the gut-brain axis, shows us the importance of the microbiome in mental health. With a decrease in your microbiome's microbiology, you are more susceptible to developing conditions like anxiety, depression, and chronic stress.

How to Keep Your Microbiome Healthy

Maintaining a healthy microbiome is very beneficial when it comes to your overall well-being. We have already looked at its diverse benefits, but here are some tips that you could use to nurture and support your microbiome.

- You must eat a balanced diet that is rich in fiber, fruits, vegetables, whole grains, and fermented foods like kefir, sauerkraut, and yogurt. All of these foods are important as they provide nourishment to the gut bacteria. Note that certain foods that digest early on in your digestive system do not actually reach your microbiome. This tends to cause them to starve. Prebiotics are the food for probiotics. You must eat more prebiotic-rich foods, such as onions, leeks, garlic, asparagus, and other green, leafy vegetables. Trying to avoid antibiotics can also help support your microbiome, as these medication types are unaware of what is good and bad bacteria and wipe out all strains. You should consider taking probiotics supplements or consuming foods that are rich in probiotics to help introduce more beneficial bacteria into your gut after a course of antibiotics.

- Eliminating stress is very beneficial, as chronic stress tends to negatively impact the microbiome. You can practice certain kinds of stress reduction techniques, like mindfulness meditation and exercise. Staying hydrated also helps support mucosal crevices and helps to maintain a healthy microbiome. You must also try to limit sugar and processed food, as they tend to become very harmful to your microbiome. Limit your intake of these.

Your microbiome is a dynamic and essential part of your biology that influences your health in profound ways. By understanding its importance and taking proactive steps to help support its balance and diversity, you can promote better health, well-being, and resilience against various diseases.

Assessing the Microbiome

It isn't very common to assess one's microbiome, but over the years, certain tests have come up that help you evaluate its condition. These include:

- Metagenomic sequencing involves the sequencing of genetic material or DNA in a microbiome sample. This gives you more comprehensive information about the microbiology community and its functional potential.
- Metabolomics is a study of the small molecules that are produced by your microbiome. It helps give information about what the metabolic activities of the microbiota are.
- Microbiome profiling kits are commercial kits now available. They allow specialized you to collect stool samples at home and then send them to a lab for microbial analysis.

If you are interested in testing your microbiome for health reasons, you can speak to your healthcare provider to find out about any specialized testing. This area is rapidly advancing and resources are coming up quickly.

As we conclude this chapter, remember that understanding your health is the only way to take that first step. You now have all the information regarding health and how you can assess the levels. However, taking action to improve your health requires motivation. In the next chapter, we're going to explore strategies that will help ignite your passion for healthy aging, turning knowledge into the driving force behind your journey. Let's harness the knowledge we have gained and use it as fuel for an extraordinary journey toward a healthier and more fulfilling future.

3

UNLEASHING MOTIVATION

> *You are never too old to set another goal or to dream a new dream.*
>
> — C.S. LEWIS

What exactly is motivation? To put it simply, motivation is the driving force behind every action and behavior. It's sort of like the inner spark within us that compels us to pursue our goals. Without motivation, we would be aimless and without any will or drive to do anything. In this chapter, we are going to explore the psychology of motivation, understand what it is, why it's essential, and how it works.

WHY IS MOTIVATION IMPORTANT?

Motivation is the cornerstone of personal growth and achievement. It is the fuel that helps propel us forward, even when we are faced with dire challenges and obstacles. Without motivation, it's challenging to initiate change, overcome inertia, or even sustain efforts over time. Motivation is crucial when it comes to driving your behavior and achieving goals (Cherry, 2023).

Motivation offers a range of benefits, which include:

- the empowerment of working toward your aspirations with dedication and perseverance
- being more productive and efficient so that you can accomplish tasks and meet your deadlines
- improved well-being, as you have a great sense of purpose and the will to find happiness; with this, you are more likely to experience fulfillment and satisfaction in your life

Motivation is a very important aspect of life, and there are several ways to obtain it. For example:

- Extrinsic motivation arises from external factors like rewards, recognition, or praise. While external influences can provide a temporary boost to your motivation, they may not sustain a long-term commitment.

- Intrinsic motivation, on the other hand, comes from within, but it is more driven by your satisfaction, sense of purpose, or the joy of the activity itself. This type of motivation is important when it comes to lasting change and meaningful growth.
- Self-motivation is the ability to generate and sustain motivation. This revolves around setting clear goals, fostering a growth mindset, and understanding your values.

Without it, severe consequences can occur both in your personal and professional aspects of life. These include:

- You will have a lack of goal pursuit, where you do not have the energy or desire to work toward any goal.
- You will find it very difficult to finish projects and take on the challenge of finding and getting involved in new opportunities, which will keep your productivity very low.
- You will experience a low energy level and decreased enthusiasm since motivation contributes to enthusiasm and a positive outlook on life.
- You will not persevere through any challenges or setbacks; in fact, you will give up in the face of adversity.

- It will have a negative emotional impact, and you may begin to develop conditions like anxiety and even depression. Your relationships will also be affected as you withdraw from social activities, which leads to strained connections with family and friends.
- You will not be able to take care of yourself health-wise. You will not exercise, care about proper nutrition, or look after your well-being. You will neglect your physical and mental health, which can lead to various health issues.

This is why motivation is so important. It plays such a significant role in healthy aging by influencing various aspects of your physical, mental, and emotional well-being. Let's take a closer look at why it's important to have motivation to ensure healthy aging.

The role of motivation in healthy aging is that as we age, it becomes very important to maintain good physical and mental health, adopt an adaptive mindset as life continuously changes, and pursue a fulfilling lifestyle. With motivation, you will be more likely to adopt and maintain healthy habits like regular exercise, eating a balanced diet, and ensuring that you get adequate sleep. All these habits are very important when it comes to maintaining physical health as we age. Staying mentally active and engaged is also vital when it comes to healthy aging.

Motivation will encourage you to seek out exciting experiences, take up new hobbies, and engage in those lifelong learning skills and techniques that all come together to help keep your mind sharp. Motivation also helps you cope with life's challenges, which include health setbacks and losses. It fosters resilience and the ability to adapt to changes, which are very important for your emotional well-being in your senior years. With motivation, you tend to maintain a more active social life compared to those without it. With social engagement, you already have better mental health, as there are fewer moments when feelings of isolation creep up, and a sense of purpose in your life offers fulfillment and satisfaction.

Motivation will help you pursue your personal goals and aspirations, whether they involve creative pursuits, volunteering, or even traveling, all of this contributes to your overall life satisfaction. Motivation is what helps us stay alive and live as though we are human beings. Without it, we are just mindless drones, carrying on each day and waiting for the end. Motivation is the foundation that leads to a strong and healthy body and mind.

Now it's time to move on to the next part of this chapter, which deals with mindfulness. Motivation, teamed with mindfulness, makes for a very powerful individual.

MINDFULNESS PRACTICES

Mindfulness is a very powerful tool that is necessary for fostering and sustaining motivation. It is all about being mentally present and in the moment without harboring any judgments or negative thoughts. This state of mind is especially relevant when it comes to healthy aging. Let's look into this in more detail (*What Is Mindfulness?*, 2020).

What Is Mindfulness?

Mindfulness is a mental practice that is done to help one learn how to pay focused and non-judgmental attention to the present moment. It helps you become aware of your thoughts, feelings, and bodily sensations without trying to change them.

You may ask the question, "What exactly does mindfulness have to do with healthy aging, and how does it benefit me?" Well, mindfulness is closely related to healthy aging, as it can have various positive effects on your mental, physical, and emotional well-being.

- You can reduce stress levels by promoting relaxation while reducing your reactivity to stressful situations.
- You also get to improve your emotional regulation while reducing symptoms of anxiety and depression.

- Mindfulness has also been linked to better cognitive function, which includes memory and attention.
- With mindfulness, you develop greater resilience in the face of life's challenges.
- There are also the benefits of pain management, where you can develop a greater tolerance while reducing the perception of pain and improving your overall comfort and quality of life.
- Mindfulness also helps foster self-awareness and self-acceptance, which gives you the knowledge to obtain a deeper understanding of your values, priorities, and life's purpose. This leads to a more fulfilling and meaningful life.
- With mindfulness, your relationships are also improved, as communication and empathy are enhanced.
- Mindfulness meditation techniques have also been shown to improve your quality of sleep. As we age, sleep disturbances become more common, and mindfulness is one basic and natural method that can help you address issues like insomnia.
- Learning to live in the moment is very important when it comes to reducing symptoms of anxiety and depression. This is mainly because, with mental health issues on the horizon, mindfulness is a valuable tool that allows you to stop worrying about the future or things that are out of your control. You learn to be in the moment,

appreciating all that you are capable of doing right now, as well as what you are experiencing in this particular moment.

How to Cultivate Mindfulness

Meditation is a very common mindfulness practice that involves sitting quietly, focusing on your breath, sensations, a thought, or a specific object and gently bringing your mind back to the focal point whenever it wanders. Let's look at a brief guided meditation practice that you could try incorporating into your daily morning routine.

Guided Meditation Practice to Develop Mindfulness

Find a quiet and comfortable room that is free of distractions. Use a cushion or a yoga mat and place it on the floor. Sit comfortably in a posture that you know will keep you aware but is not so comfortable that you will fall asleep. Select a point of focus. Many choose the breath as their point of focus, but you can also choose an object that you can place in front of your body.

- Close your eyes and begin by taking deep, calming breaths.
- Focus on the air coming in through your nose, settling in your lungs, filling your chest, and slowly exiting through your mouth.
- Keep your mind focused on the way your body feels with each breath that enters and leaves.

- Focus on breathing in and breathing out. If any thoughts are coming into your mind, allow them to move in, but do not latch onto any of them. Acknowledge that you have thoughts coming in, but if they are negative, do not stop your meditation practice, acknowledge the thought, or emotion, and then let it go... like passing clouds on a sunny day. Acknowledge that you have gone through a negative thought and allowed it to move freely away without latching onto it.
- Continue focusing on your breathing.
- Breathe deeply—breathing in, breathing out, and breathing in again as you keep your mind focused on your breath. If not your breath, you are focused on the object in front of you.
- Once you feel that you are ready, slowly begin to focus on your breathing again.
- Breathe in and breathe out deeply as you open your eyes and bring your awareness back to your surroundings.

Mindful breathing is when you pay attention to your breath as you inhale and exhale slowly and deliberately. It is a very simple yet effective way to practice mindfulness, and you can incorporate it into your daily meditation technique, which we have looked at previously, especially if you aren't very fond of using a different focal point.

You can also engage in everyday activities with full awareness. This is where you put yourself 100% into each process. For example, if you are eating food, you should practice mindful eating, where you savor each bite of food. If you are going on a walk, you should practice mindful walking, where you pay attention to every step that you take, as well as what is going on around you.

The link between mindfulness and motivation is that they are interconnected. With mindfulness, your focus and concentration are improved, which makes it easier for you to stay committed to your goals and maintain that motivation. Mindfulness also helps reduce procrastination by helping you become more aware of the present moment, which makes it less tempting to put things off.

Motivation and mindfulness go hand in hand, as they both help to reduce your stress and anxiety levels. Remember that mindfulness will always help you create a more conducive mental environment for your motivation to thrive. Being aware of yourself and whatever is going on around you is a side effect of mindfulness. It encourages you to reflect inwardly and gives you the benefit of developing awareness of your values. This helps you align your goals with your values, thus enhancing intrinsic motivation.

To summarize, mindfulness will boost motivation by increasing your self-awareness, reducing the number of distractions that go on around you and in your mind, and enhancing emotional regulation and resilience. Mindfulness also helps to mitigate procrastination, improve goal setting, reduce stress, and enhance decision-making skills. By incorporating mindfulness practices into your daily life, you can cultivate a mindset that is more conducive to maintaining motivation and achieving your desired outcomes. As you incorporate mindfulness practices, you can contribute to a holistic approach to healthy aging that addresses your physical, mental, and emotional aspects of well-being. As you foster motivation and promote well-being, mindfulness can help you age with grace while maintaining a high quality of life as you navigate the challenges and opportunities of later years.

You must incorporate mindfulness into your daily routine, as this is very valuable in maintaining your motivation for healthy aging. Not only will it help you stay present but it will also help you adapt to change and pursue your goals with a renewed sense of purpose and enthusiasm.

TECHNIQUES FOR SETTING AND ACHIEVING GOALS

Now let's look at setting and achieving goals. What does this have to do with healthy aging? Goal-setting is a very powerful activity when it comes to maintaining motivation. Whether you have a well-defined goal or one that is still in its development stages, you have chosen a direction to move toward the path of being active. This helps keep you focused and driven, which is going to help build your motivation.

The Importance of Goal-Setting

Goal-setting helps provide you with clarity about what you want to achieve in your life and helps you stay focused on your desired outcomes. Setting goals also helps create a sense of purpose and motivation, driving you forward and making you choose a course of action as you strive toward achieving what you have set out for.

Goals are measurable, or at least you should make them measurable, and this will allow you to track your progress and celebrate your successes along the way. Your goals should also hold you accountable for your actions and decisions, as it makes it less likely for you to procrastinate or lose sight of your aspirations. Basically, without a goal, you are an aimless individual. Not knowing what you want to do with your life can have a devastating impact on your mental health and well-being. The reason why goal-setting is important is because it gives you a sense of purpose and the will to keep living. Without any goals, you would live from day to day with no enjoyment or sense of fulfillment from your life.

Setting SMART Goals

You have already seen two terms that have resonated throughout this book. One is that your goals should be accountable, and the other is measurable. Now let's look at the SMART goal-setting system, which gives you more details and insight. SMART stands for:

- **S**pecific: All of your goals must be precise. They should be clear about what you want to accomplish, who is involved, where it will happen, and why it's important. It's important that you understand and see what your goal is instead of being crowded with unnecessary information. Compare "I want to be healthy," to "I want to exercise for 10 minutes a day and eat a healthy lunch afterward."
- **M**easurable: You should be able to acknowledge your progress and determine when the goal has been achieved. This helps you stay in charge by knowing where you are in completing your goals, which directly affects your motivation levels. As you see your progress, you will feel more motivated to complete your goals. Compare "I must be fit" to "I will be able to lift a 5-pound weight by the end of this month."
- **A**chievable: Every individual is only capable of so much. For this reason, ensure that the goal you have set out for yourself is one that is realistic and

attainable. It should be challenging but within your capabilities of achieving. Setting goals that are too difficult or demanding and out of your capability will decrease your motivation to get it completed. Compare "I must be able to look like Mr. Olympia at the end of this," to "I must be able to get stronger than I currently am, moving from a 2-pound weight to a 5-pound weight at the end of week four."

- **R**elevant: Anyone can come up with any kind of goal, but the difference is that your goals should not be just any random thing. It has to be meaningful and relevant to you. It should align with your objectives and values. Compare "I need to live longer," to "I need to increase my fitness levels and enhance my mental health using healthy aging tips and advice to improve my longevity."
- **T**ime-Bound: You should always set a timeframe for your goals. By having a deadline, there will be a sense of urgency, which helps you prioritize your actions and complete your goals. Compare "I must become strong" to "I must become more flexible to reach my toes while stretching my hamstrings at the end of the second week of training."

IDENTIFYING AND ALIGNING WITH YOUR VALUES

When we think of values, we understand that they are the deeply held beliefs and principles that guide our behavior and decisions. Aligning your goals with your values will significantly boost your motivation, as it provides you with a sense of fulfillment. The Shwartz Values Theory identifies several values, which include self-direction, benevolence, achievement, and others. Let's look at how aligning with your values can boost your motivation (Schwartz, 2011).

- There is increased meaning and purpose since your goals align with your values, and this can motivate you even further.
- Since values act as a source of resilience, especially when you are faced with challenges, you know that you are working toward something that aligns with what you find worthy. This will help keep you persistent as you move forward.
- Goals that align with your values are more likely to tap into intrinsic motivation. This means that you will enjoy the process and find personal satisfaction in achieving the goal.
- Your values will serve as a compass for decision-making, when you align your actions with your values, it becomes easier to make choices that support your goals.

- By aligning your actions with your values, you will feel more authentic and consistent as you pursue your goals. This will increase your motivation, guiding you to stay on track.

Tips for Aligning With Your Values

- Reflect on your values as you take time to identify and clarify what they are. Try to find out what principles are most important to you.
- Review your existing goals and see how well they align with your values. You can always adjust them as needed.
- Focus on pursuing goals that resonate with your values and contribute to your sense of purpose.
- By periodically reflecting on your values and how they relate to your goals, you can stay aligned and motivated.
- Share your values and goals with friends or a support network so they can provide encouragement and help you stay on track.

Incorporating all of these strategies into your goal-setting process will help lead to a more meaningful and motivating pursuit, which will ultimately contribute to a fulfilling and purpose-driven life.

What Gives Life Meaning and Purpose

If you are wondering about life and what gives it meaning and purpose, this can open a doorway to information that will profoundly influence your motivation.

The purpose of life is one question that many people have. In fact, scholars, philosophers, and individuals have pondered the answer to this question for centuries. The answer always came out differently. Some find their path in different fields: religion, personal relationships, achievements, and other things important to them.

Discovering the purpose of your life can be a game-changer for you. It can give a new sense of direction and a goal to work toward. This new path will be a helpful source of motivation, guiding and urging you forward.

How to Find More Purpose in Life

- Reflect on what truly excites you. What makes you feel fulfilled with life or a certain activity or task?
- Identify what your values are. What are the principles that guide your decisions?
- Sometimes your purpose does not only involve your life but others as well. Help others.
- As you embrace challenges, you may realize that your purpose emerges from overcoming adversity.

- Define specific and meaningful goals that align with your purpose.
- Look within and discover what type of individual you are. What makes you happy? What interests you? What should happen or involve you to help you be fulfilled in life?

Once you find purpose in your life, it makes it much easier to grasp hold of that motivation to ensure that you are going to commit to a healthy lifestyle plan, changing the habits you once had that led to a detrimental health and aging process. Finding your purpose here can be anything from learning how to age gracefully' not wanting to fall victim to a health condition; not wanting to lose your health, freedom, mobility; and so much more. By learning about healthy living and healthy aging, you can even move forward and go out there to help others move onto this path where they too can lead healthier lives, aging as though nothing had changed as they moved from the adult to senior phase of life.

Positive Psychology

This is a beacon of life that illuminates the path toward motivation and healthy aging. It mainly focuses on making life more fulfilling. By embracing positive psychology, we can all thrive as we age. Here are some key concepts related to positive psychology.

- Optimism: This isn't just about trying to see the bright side in every situation; it's about believing that good things can come to pass, even in those stressful, challenging, and depressing moments of life. This way of looking at life and moving through it can boost your motivation, urging you to move forward, no matter what kind of situation you are in.
- Resilience: This is more like a superpower in our world. Very few have the ability to walk out of a stressful and challenging situation with a smile on their face and their back still straight. Resilience is the ability to bounce back after a setback. The ability to get back up after being knocked down, again and again When it comes to healthy aging, this is a very valuable trait, as it helps you stay focused and motivated even in the face of adversity.
- Growth mindset: This is the belief that you can develop and grow your abilities over time. You understand that you will never be able to stop improving. As you age, you still have the capacity to learn new things, adapt, and advance. This is a key ingredient in staying motivated as you age.

Positivity is what inspires us and helps us move forward. Without it, the world would be full of drones, no one seeing the colors that surround them except black, white, and gray. But it doesn't have to be this way. We can change and break the rules of aging, knowing that we don't have to follow the ways of the past and that we can fight the natural process through natural means. With a positive mindset, all things are possible, especially healthy aging.

As we conclude, remember that your journey to a healthier and more vibrant life through exercise is just around the corner. Before we move into the next chapter, steel your nerves. Wrap the knowledge of motivation, a positive mindset, and the ability to adapt, grow, evolve, and succeed around you with a boost of encouragement and motivation. You are armed and ready to take the next step. Get ready to face the next part of this journey with enthusiasm and determination.

MAKE A DIFFERENCE WITH YOUR REVIEW

UNLOCK THE POWER OF GENEROSITY

> "Money can't buy happiness, but giving it away can."
>
> — FREDDIE MERCURY

People who give without expectation live longer, happier lives and make more money. So if we've got a shot at that during our time together, darn it, I'm gonna try..

To make that happen, I have a question for you...

Would you help someone you've never met, even if you never got credit for it?

Who is this person you ask? They are like you. Or, at least, like you used to be. Less experienced, wanting to make a difference, and needing help, but not sure where to look.

Our mission is to make Discover Healthy Aging and Longevity accessible to everyone. Everything we do stems from that mission. And, the only way for us to accomplish that mission is by reaching...well...everyone.

This is where you come in. Most people do, in fact, judge a book by its cover (and its reviews). So here's my ask on behalf of a struggling, aging, adult you've never met:

Please help that future Super Ager by leaving this book a review.

Your gift costs no money and less than 60 seconds to make real, but can change a fellow Journey Ager's life forever. Your review could help…

...one more small businesses provide for their community.

...one more entrepreneur support their family.

...one more employee get meaningful work.

..one more client transform their life.

...one more dream come true.

To get that 'feel good' feeling and help this person for real, all you have to do is...and it takes less than 60 seconds...

leave a review.

Simply scan the QR code below to leave your review:

If you feel good about helping a faceless healthy ager, you are my kind of person. Welcome to the club. You're one of us.

I'm that much more excited to help you achieve Healthier Aging faster and easier than you can possibly imagine. You'll love the strategies I'm about to share in the coming chapters.

Thank you from the bottom of my heart. Now, back to our regularly scheduled program-ming.

- Your biggest fan, B B Joseph

4

REVITALIZING THROUGH EXERCISE

> *Movement is a medicine for creating change in a person's physical, emotional, and mental states.*
>
> — CAROL WELCH

It's time to move into the active part of this journey. There is transformative power in exercise when it comes to healthy aging. At the end of this chapter, you will have a much deeper understanding of why exercise is vital for your well-being, as well as the various types of exercises available, their benefits, and how you can safely incorporate them into your daily routine.

It has been a stereotype that people over the age of 50 can't do much activity with their bodies, as aging has already begun to take a toll and any sort of rigorous or high-impact exercise will cause more harm than good for their bodies. There are quite a lot of misconceptions concerning this, and it invades society and makes people believe conflicting information. This is especially wrong since it concerns the health and well-being of the human body.

Let's move into the topic to find out why it's so important.

THE VALUE OF EXERCISE

Exercise is crucial, and some of the reasons include (*Benefits of Physical Activity*, 2021):

Physical Health Benefits

Exercising regularly helps to keep your body strong and improves your cardiovascular health while reducing the risk of chronic diseases and directly promoting longevity.

Your arteries, organs, and other body parts are severely impacted by all the changes that are going on inside of you. Not participating in any form of exercise can make the effects of aging much worse, and as a senior, you will feel them more harshly. As you exercise, all of these issues are diminished. With exercise, you can eradicate the physical impact of aging.

Let's look at Sally, a retiree who started lifting weights in her 60s. Initially, she struggled to lift even light dumbbells, but with time and dedication, she became stronger, enabling her to carry groceries, play with her grandkids, and enjoy hiking trips well into her 70s.

Mental Health Benefits

Exercise is the best natural mood booster and stress reliever there is. Exercising regularly comes with the release of dopamine, which is the body's natural stress reliever and mood regulator. This is not the only benefit that your mind receives from exercise. Alongside this, as you regularly participate in exercise and other physical routines, your body tends to become stronger and more flexible. With the acknowledgment that you aren't going through the regular stages of aging, you will feel much happier and more confident. Noticing that your body is stronger, and your posture is the same as that of a 30-year-old will also help boost your confidence and make you stand up tall. With these benefits, your mind and mental health are improved and enhanced daily.

Seeing the benefits of your exercise also tends to keep you motivated and happier. We have already gone through the information about why you need to be motivated and positive throughout your day. By participating in exercise daily, you will not need to work hard to incorporate these concepts into your lifestyle. Tave, in his late 80s, joined a dance class for seniors. Not only did he make new friends, but he also found that dancing lifted his spirits and helped him cope with the loss of his spouse.

Longevity

Already having a direct impact on your life—from a strong and healthy physique to a resilient and healthy mindset—exercise boosts your longevity. Consistent exercise routines add vibrant years to your life. This is not some pitch to get you to keep exercising. It is true and backed up by research (*Benefits of Physical Activity*, 2022). With exercise, there is a decreased risk of becoming obese. It also helps improve your cardiovascular health and maintain your blood sugar levels. Exercise also helps to prevent certain cancers from developing, as well as enabling and enhancing processes within the body, for example, homeostasis, the nervous system, and the body's ability to attack and prevent disease.

Let us consider the case of Marge, who celebrated her 80th birthday with a hike up a mountain. She attributed her longevity and vitality to her lifelong commitment to staying physically active through activities like gardening and daily walks.

Types of Exercises and Their Benefits

This is not about the grueling workouts that most people are aware of. This is about enjoyable activities that can fit into any lifestyle, and you can begin them no matter what your fitness levels are or at any age. Let's look at them in detail (*The 4 Most Important Types of Exercise - Harvard Health*, 2017):

Cardiovascular and Aerobic Exercises

These types of exercises improve your heart and lung health, as well as increase your stamina, burn calories, and help with weight management. These exercises also reduce the risk of chronic diseases like stroke, heart disease, and diabetes.

Some examples of cardiovascular and aerobic exercise include running, jogging, cycling, swimming, dancing, brisk walking, and more.

Strength Training Exercises

Building muscle mass increases your metabolism, enhances your overall strength and endurance, and improves bone density. These exercises also help with weight management and injury prevention.

Some examples include weightlifting, using resistance bands for some exercises, body weight exercises, and machine workouts. These include push-ups, squats, lunges, and so on.

Flexibility and Stretching

These exercises improve your joints' range of motion, reduce muscle tension, and enhance your body's posture while decreasing the risk of injuries. These exercises are also very good for relaxing and reducing stress.

Some examples include yoga, Pilates, static stretching, dynamic stretching, and mobility exercises.

Balance and Stability Exercises

These help improve your coordination, prevent falling, enhance your core strength, and help you maintain functional independence. This is very important for your senior years.

Some examples of these types of exercises include tai chi and chi gong balance, stability balls, and specific yoga poses.

High-Intensity Interval Training (HIIT)

HIIT improves cardiovascular fitness, burns calories efficiently, boosts your metabolism, and can be time-efficient. These exercises also help with weight loss and muscle toning. They are recommended for you only if you are strong and flexible enough.

Some exercise examples include short bursts of intense activity followed by a brief rest or lower-intensity periods. If you would like to try high-intensity interval training for low fitness levels, you could always try walking and then jogging for a few seconds, or you could jog for a few seconds and then switch to fast running. Make sure to start jogging and stop running at different intervals.

Functional Training Exercises

These enhance your overall strength, mobility, and stability, as they make it much easier for you to perform daily tasks while reducing the risk of injuries.

Some examples include those that may involve everyday movements like lunges, squats, and kettlebell swings.

Mind-Body Exercise

This combines physical movement with mental focus and relaxation to promote stress reduction, improve mindfulness, and strengthen the mind-body connection.

Some examples include yoga, tai chi ,chi gong, and Pilates.

Low-Impact Exercise

This is the most common exercise suggested for aging adults. It is gentle on the joints and suitable for those with joint problems or injuries. It still offers cardiovascular benefits and calorie burning. Some of these types include aerobics, stationary cycling, and elliptical training. Note that other types of exercises, including Pilates and body-weight exercises, swimming, and rowing can also fall under low-impact exercises.

The Benefits

There are quite a few benefits of exercising, and these include:

- boosting your stamina, strengthening your heart, and providing an energy surplus for daily life
- strengthening your bones and muscles, and ligaments, making you stronger, preventing frailty and falls
- reducing the risk of accidents and improving your overall quality of life
- improving and enhancing your range of motion, reducing muscle tension, and promoting relaxation

WARM-UPS AND STRETCHING

One basic mistake many people make when it comes to physical activity is not warming up. Before any sort of exercise routine, you must warm up to prevent injuries while training. This, however, is not the only benefit of warming up. Let's look into this in more detail and learn why you need to stretch before exercise.

Warming up is also very important to help increase blood flow to your muscles, making them more pliable and less prone to strain. With proper warm-ups, your muscles and joint flexibility are enhanced, which leads to better athletic performance and range of motion. Your heart rate is elevated gradually, which prepares your cardiovascular system for more intense activity. It also helps activate your nervous system and improve your coordination and balance. Warming up also mentally prepares you for exercise and allows you to focus while setting your intentions for the upcoming activities.

Let's take a look at a few warm-up exercises you can do at home.

Arm Circles

- Stand with your feet shoulder-width apart.
- Extend your arms straight out to your sides.
- Begin by making small circles with your arm, rotating them in a clockwise direction.
- Gradually increase the size of the circles.
- After 15 to 20 seconds, stop and then reverse the direction of your circles.
- Continue in this motion for one to three minutes.

Leg Swings

- Stand near a wall or sturdy chair for support or balance.
- Swing one leg forward and backward in a controlled manner.
- Hold on to the wall if you feel that you cannot balance on one leg.

- Perform 10 to 15 swings with one leg before stopping and switching positions with the other.
- Perform the same number of swings with the other leg.

Cat-Cow Stretch

- Begin by getting down on your hands and knees in a tabletop position on a soft carpet or yoga mat.
- Inhale as you begin to arch your back, lifting your head and tailbone. This is known as the cow position.
- Exhale as you round your back, tucking your chin and tailbone. This is known as the cat position.
- Repeat this motion for one to three minutes.

Quadriceps Stretch

- Stand tall with your feet hip-width apart beside a wall, which you can place one hand against for balance.
- Bend one knee and bring your heel toward your buttocks.
- Hold your ankle with your hand as you gently pull your heel closer.
- Keep your knees close and your torso upright.
- Hold the position for 15 to 30 seconds on each leg.

Always keep in mind that it's important to customize your warm-up routines based on the activity and needs you have. You should also gradually increase the intensity of your warm-up to match the demands of your exercise routines.

COOL-DOWN STRETCHES

Cool-down stretches are just as important as warm-up exercises, as they assist your body in preventing injury after a workout. It also promotes recovery, prevents dizziness, and improves flexibility, mental relaxation, and flexibility. It's always advisable that you do specific cool-down stretches to target the muscles you worked out during your exercise routine. Some of these stretches include:

Child's Pose for Back and Hips

- Get down on your knees with your hands in a tabletop position.
- Sit back on your heels as you lower your chest toward the floor.
- Extend your arms forward and rest your forehead on the ground.
- Hold this position for 30 to 60 seconds as you focus on deep breathing.

Seated Hamstring Stretch

- Sit on the floor with your legs extended straight out in front of you.
- Hinge at your hips as you reach for your toes with both hands.
- Keep your back straight and avoid rounding your spine during this movement.
- Hold the stretch for 15 to 30 seconds as you feel a gentle pull in your hamstrings.

Always keep in mind that you should perform your cool-down stretches gently as you hold each stretch without forcing or bouncing your body.

You should always be comfortable and in a relaxed position as you breathe deeply throughout the stretches.

Note that cooling down properly is just as important as warming up to maintain flexibility and prevent injuries.

RANGE OF MOTION AND MOBILITY

This is a very crucial part of maintaining your physical functionality as you age. Range of motion is the term that is used to refer to how much movement your joints can achieve in various directions. It is the key to maintaining flexibility and the capability of performing day-to-day tasks without any discomfort.

On the other hand, mobility encompasses your overall ability to move freely. It's more about the coordination of your muscles, joints, and nervous system to come together and produce efficient and pain-free movements. Let's look at some practical exercises and tips that you could use to enhance your range of motion and mobility.

Before engaging in any type of exercise, always remember to warm up.

Neck Rotations

- Stand up or sit down.
- Relax your shoulders.
- Slowly begin to turn your head to the right as you bring your chin toward your shoulder.
- Hold this position for a few seconds as you feel a gentle stretch.
- Turn your head to the center and then repeat on the left side.
- Do this for 8 to 10 repetitions on each side.

Shoulder Circles

- Stand tall with your feet shoulder-width apart.
- Slowly circle your shoulders forward as you make big circles.
- Repeat the motion in the opposite position.

Hip Flexor Stretch

- Begin by kneeling on the floor with one knee.
- Keep your back straight as you gently push your hips forward.
- You should begin to feel a stretch in your front hip.
- Hold this position for 20 to 30 seconds on each side.

Quad Stretch

- Begin by standing on one leg as you hold onto a chair or a wall for balance.
- Bend your knee as you bring your heel toward your buttocks.
- Grab your ankles with your hand and gently pull your heel closer.
- Hold this position for 20 to 30 seconds on each leg.

Calf Stretch

- Stand tall facing a wall.
- Your hands should be shoulder-width apart.
- Step with one foot back as you press the heel into the floor.
- You should begin to feel a stretch in your calf muscle.

- Hold this position for 20 to 30 seconds on each side.
- Repeat these 5 to 10 times.

Spinal Twist

- Sit on the floor with your legs extended in front of you.
- Bend one knee and cross it over the opposite leg.
- Place your opposite hand on the bent knee and gently twist your torso toward that side.
- Hold this position for 20 to 30 seconds on each side.
- Repeat these 5 to 10 times.

Ankle Circles

- Sit on a chair with your feet flat on the floor.
- Begin by lifting one foot off the ground and rotating your ankle in a circular motion.
- Do these 10 to 15 times in one direction before switching to the other.
- Repeat this motion on your other leg.

Toe Touches

- Sit on the floor with your legs straight in front of you.
- Slowly begin to bend forward from your hips as you reach your hand down toward your toes.
- Do not force the stretch.
- Go only as far as is comfortable for your body.
- Hold the position for 20 to 30 seconds.
- Repeat this motion five to eight times.

Deep Breathing

- Sit down or lie down comfortably on a soft carpet or yoga mat.
- Begin by taking slow, deep diaphragmatic
- breaths in through your nose and out through your mouth.
- Focus on expanding your lungs and rib cage with each breath.
- This helps relax your muscles and improve your overall mobility.
- Take as many breaths as you feel comfortable.

For range-of-motion and mobility exercises, you could also try out some low-impact water aerobics, tai chi, ball exercises, yoga poses, and simple resistance band exercises.

THE ROLES OF CARDIO AND STRENGTH TRAINING

Cardiovascular health and fitness alongside strength training are the two pillars of a well-rounded exercise routine. Not only are you targeting external body parts but also your internal structure. Let's look at a few practical examples that provide a deeper look into the significance of each of these pillars.

Cardio targets your heart, lungs, and circulatory system. The activities here keep your breathing and heart rate elevated for an extended period. Some of the benefits include:

- strengthening your heart muscle and making it more efficient at pumping blood and oxygen throughout the body
- reducing the risk of heart disease while improving overall cardiovascular health
- helping to burn calories and support weight loss and weight management
- increasing your stamina and endurance, which allows you to engage in daily activities without feeling tired easily

There are different types of cardio, which include running cycling, swimming, brisk walking, dancing, aerobics, and other exercises. Experts recommend at least 150 minutes of moderate-intensity aerobic exercise or 75 minutes of vigorous-intensity aerobic exercise per week for optimum cardiovascular health (Laskowski, 2023).

Strength training, on the other hand, is also known as resistance training, and it focuses on building and strengthening your muscles by using resistance like weights, resistance bands, or even your own body weight. Some of the benefits include:

- helping to build and maintain muscle mass, which is very important for functional strength and stability in daily life
- boosting your metabolism, which helps to decrease the amount of fat tissue in your body
- promoting your bone density, which reduces the risk of osteoporosis
- strengthening your muscles around the joints, which can help alleviate joint pain while reducing the risk of injuries as you move

There are different types of strength training that can be done using free weights machines, resistance bands, or body-weight exercises like push-ups, squats, and more. When it comes to the frequency, you should always aim to do at least two to three times of training each week.

When it comes to the complementary roles, increased endurance and stamina allow you to perform strength training exercises more effectively. For example, if you were doing a bout of strength exercises, better cardiovascular fitness will help you maintain the intensity and complete the routine. Cardio and strength training also offer a very comprehensive approach to your overall health. Cardio targets your health while strength training addresses your muscles and bone health, which reduces the risk of chronic diseases while enhancing your body's health and longevity.

Other benefits include:

- injury prevention, as both come together by improving your muscle imbalances and supporting your joint instability while engaging in intense cardio activities
- managing your weight, as it burns calories throughout the workout with cardio exercises, and strength training builds muscles, which continue to burn fat at rest

Cardio Exercises to Try

Before you begin any type of exercise, always remember to warm up. Also, remember to start at your fitness level and then increase the intensity or duration of the exercise to avoid overexertion and reduce the risk of injury (Lane, 2021).

- Running is a classic cardio exercise and can be done outdoors or on a treadmill.
- Cycling on a stationary bike or riding outdoors is a low impact yet effective way to boost your heart rate while strengthening your leg muscles.
- Jumping rope is another efficient cardio exercise that can be done anywhere. It is also great for improving your coordination and agility.
- Swimming is a low-impact exercise that targets a full-body workout that is gentle on your joints and yet effective.
- Rowing machines also provide a great workout while engaging both your upper and lower body.
- Aerobic dances are grateful for their cardio elements, as they provide you with an engaging and effective workout.
- Stair climbing is a simple but challenging work cardio workout that also targets your leg muscles and improves your endurance.

Some cardio exercises that you could try at home include:

Jumping Jacks

- Start with your feet together and your arms at your sides.
- Jump while simultaneously spreading your legs apart, at the same time raising your arms over your head.

- Jump back to the starting position.
- Continue with this motion for 30 to 45 seconds.

High Knees

- Begin by standing in place with your feet hip-width apart.
- Lift one knee up as high as you can while driving the opposite arm up.
- Alternate rapidly between both legs as if jogging in place.

Mountain Climbers

- Begin by getting in a plank position with your hands directly under your shoulder and your body in a straight line on the floor.
- Stay in this position, ensuring that your back is straight, not hunched or sagging.
- Alternate as you bring your left knee toward your chest first, then return it back to position, and then bring your right leg toward your chest before bringing it back to your starting position.
- Engage your core with deep breathing and maintaining a brisk but steady pace.

Strength Training Exercises to Try

Let's investigate some simple exercises now (Lane, 2021):

Body-Weight Squats

- Stand up straight with your feet shoulder-width apart.
- Your back should be straight with your shoulders back.
- Lower your body by bending your knees and hips.
- Hold this position for three to five seconds.
- Push through your heels to return to the starting position.
- Repeat 10 to 15 times.
- Perform three sets.

Push-Ups

- Start by getting into a plank position with your hands placed shoulder-width apart.
- Lower your body by bending your elbows until your chest is close to the floor.
- Stay in this position for one to two seconds before pushing yourself up to the starting position.
- Your back, shoulders, and legs should be aligned.
- Do not sag or arch your back.

- You can modify this exercise by doing knee push-ups if you have back issues or pain or if you find it's too difficult for you.
- Perform three sets with 10 to 12 repetitions of this exercise.

Plank

- Begin by lying face down with your forearms on the ground and your elbows directly under your shoulders.
- Lift your body off the ground as you keep your body in a straight line from your head to your heels.
- Hold this position for as long as you can, aiming for at least 30 to 60 seconds.

Lunges

- Begin by standing with your feet placed together.
- Take a medium step forward with one foot and lower your body until both knees are bent at 90-degree angles.
- Hold this position for two to three seconds before pushing off with the front foot to return to your starting position.
- Alternate between each leg and aim for 12 to 15 repetitions per leg and three sets.

Tricep Dips

- Start by sitting on the edge of a stable chair or bench with your hands gripping the edge.
- Slide your buttocks off the chair and bend your elbows to lower your body using your arms for the movement.
- Slowly begin to push back up to your starting position after two to three seconds.
- Perform 10 to 12 repetitions and three sets.

Always remember to perform your warm-up exercises before your strength training routines and cool down with some light stretches after you have completed the activities.

Exercises Outside the Gym

Exercising indoors, at home, or in the gym frequently can get a little boring and demotivating. There is a fix for this where you can get your daily dose of exercise outside. Some of the activities that you could try include (Day, 2022):

- Take a brisk walk in the park or along scenic trails.
- Whether on a track or through a nature reserve, you can try out some running.

- Explore different trails and elevate your heart rate with nature hiking.
- You could also try riding a bike through your local neighborhood or on a dedicated bike path.
- You can try rollerblading at your favorite park.
- Jumping rope on a flat surface is another great way to work out.
- You could practice outdoor yoga in the park or at the beach.
- Tai chi is another great exercise to try outdoors.
- You could play beach volleyball to get a full-body workout.
- You could also use playground equipment to do certain exercises like pull-ups and tricep dips.
- You can go kayaking or canoeing through a serene lake or river.
- If you love the water, you could also try to do some water aerobics or swimming.
- Go outdoors and find a set of stairs or a hill to challenge yourself with uphill climbing.
- You could invite some friends over to the park and play a friendly game of frisbee.
- You could go out trail running with a group of friends or family.
- Outdoor rock climbing is another great way to get a full-body workout while exploring nature.

The major benefit of outdoor exercise is that you get to mentally unwind and de-stress as you spend time in nature.

Weightless At-Home Body Exercises

If going out to the gym or outdoors to exercise isn't really your thing, you could always stay at home and try out body-weight exercises to keep you fit and healthy instead. They are a fantastic way for you to stay active without the need for any equipment. Some of these activities that you could try include:

Squats

- Begin by standing with your feet shoulder-width apart.
- Lower your body by bending your knees (remember to not exceed a 90 degree bend at your knee) and pushing your hips back.
- Keep your back straight and your chest up.
- Hold this position for two to three seconds before returning to the starting position by pushing through your heels.
- Repeat 10 to 12 times.
- Perform two to four sets.

Bicycle Crunches

- Begin by lying down on your back with your hands behind your head.
- Lift your head and shoulders a little off the ground.
- Raise your feet slightly off the ground as you bring one knee toward your chest while simultaneously twisting your torso to bring the opposite elbow toward that knee.
- Alternate sides as though doing a pedaling motion.
- Perform 8 to 14 repetitions and two to three sets.

Supermans

- Begin by lying face down with your arms extended in front of you.
- Simultaneously, lift your arms, chest, and legs off the ground.
- Hold this position for a few seconds before lowering your body back down to your starting position.
- Repeat six to eight reps.
- Perform two to three sets.

Wall Sits

- Begin by standing with your back against a wall and your feet about hip-width apart.
- Slide down the wall until your knees are bent at a 90-degree angle.
- Hold this position for at least 30 to 60 seconds as you engage your leg muscles.
- Keep your core engaged with deep breathing.

Burpees

- Begin by standing up straight.
- In a fluid and quick motion, drop into a squat position with your hands on the ground.
- Move forward, kicking your feet back into a plank position.
- Immediately return your feet to the squat position.
- Next, explosively jump up from the squat position.
- Repeat 8 to 15 times.
- Perform two to three sets of this exercise.

You could also try push-ups, tricep dips, planks, lunges, and mountain climbers.

These are some great exercises that you could try at home to help you build strength, increase your endurance, and improve your overall fitness without going to the gym and needing all that machinery.

SELECTING AND COMMITTING TO AN EXERCISE ROUTINE

Choosing the right type of exercise routine that is designed to suit your needs, preferences, and fitness level is very important when it comes to long-term success and motivation. Let's look at a guide that will help you make the right choice.

How to Choose an Exercise Routine That Fits Your Needs

- Determine what you want to achieve with your exercise routine. Decide whether it's weight loss, muscle gain, improved cardiovascular health, stress reduction, or staying alive for longer. With a clear goal, you will be able to select your exercise routine much more easily.
- Assessing your current fitness levels will also give you an idea of where to start. You will know what level matches your abilities and what types of exercises will prevent overexertion and reduce the risk of injury.
- Decide what type of activities you enjoy. When you find the ones that you genuinely like doing, you will stay committed more easily.

- Consider a well-rounded routine that will include a variety of exercise types. This will not only prevent boredom but also ensure that you are getting a balanced approach to fitness.
- Commit to a workout schedule that will fit your daily life. Always remember that consistency will be more important than intensity. You should always start with a few days a week and gradually increase as you build endurance.
- If you are still unsure about what to decide on, you can always seek professional guidance to help create a tailored plan and teach you the proper form for your exercise routines.
- Keep track of your progress with a fitness journal to track your achievements and identify areas for improvement. You should always celebrate your successes every step of the journey. This will help you stay motivated and persistent in your exercise journey.

How to Stay Motivated

During our older years, it can be very difficult to stay motivated. Then again, with aging effects, less endurance, and low energy levels, motivation is reduced even more. However, there are some strategies that you could implement to help you stay on track. These include:

- Find someone to work out with. This could either be a friend or family member who can make workouts more enjoyable and help you keep to your workout routines.
- Set milestones where you break your long-term goals into smaller, more achievable ones.
- Celebrate each milestone as you progress. You could also try new activities. By keeping your routine fresh, it is more exciting, and this can be very encouraging.
- Use technology like fitness apps for wearables. You could also follow online communities, which can provide you with motivation to continue your exercises, help you keep track, and offer guidance.
- Reward yourself for meeting all of your fitness goals. Every time. You should also remind yourself of the benefits of the exercises, so you are motivated and encouraged to continue moving forward.

HOW TO ADVANCE TO HIGHER LEVELS OF FITNESS

If you exercise, it does not matter how much or how many days a week, eventually, you will become stronger. The exercise routines that you are currently engaging in will seem as though they are no longer as difficult or strenuous. For this reason, you will need to advance your fitness levels safely. This will help you increase and boost your strength and endurance. Some of the ways to do this include:

- Progress gradually, increasing the intensity and duration of frequency of your workouts slowly but surely. Always remember that pushing yourself too hard will lead to injuries, injuries that will derail you exercise program. You should also ensure your routine includes rest days, which allow your body to recover and adapt to the stress.
- Add resistance. For example, strength training will require you to increase the weights or the tension of the resistance bands to challenge your muscles.
- Modify your exercises to make them more challenging, like having a stability ball or performing single-leg variations of a specific exercise.
- Pay attention to your diet to support your increased activity levels. Always keep in mind that with exercise you will need to feed your muscles. They are protein-based fibers and to repair or help grow and make them stronger, you will need to incorporate more protein in your diet. Without it, your all muscle fibers will starve.

Now that you are informed on all you need to know about exercise and how to keep your body fit and healthy through activities, it's time to explore the vital connection between exercise and nutrition as we unveil how these two elements work in supporting your journey toward healthy aging. Get ready for a well-rounded approach to a vibrant life.

5

NOURISHING THROUGH NUTRITION

> *Let thy food be your medicine, and your medicine be your food.*
>
> — HIPPOCRATES

These words echo a timeless truth. There is healing power in food. It's time for us to look into the vibrant world of nutrition. We are going to uncover the profound role nutrition plays in your health and longevity. What is our goal? It's about equipping you with a deeper understanding of dietary recommendations, with a spotlight on the miraculous Mediterranean diet.

A CLOSER LOOK AT METABOLISM

During our lives, we tend to notice certain things that make us stand out. For example, we wonder why some people seem to eat anything and everything they want without gaining a single pound while others merely look at a hot dog or sandwich and their jeans feel tighter than usual. The basic reason why each person differs is because of their metabolism. To put it simply, this is the process that is used to burn calories in return for energy.

A simple way of looking at it is to think of metabolism as your body's energy factory. It is the process of converting the food you eat into fuel to assist with every body function. It is vital that you understand that energy is needed for almost every process that occurs within your body, from blinking your eyes to running a marathon. Every cell will require energy to function. However, there is one change that happens when you age: Your metabolism rate decreases as well.

As we have already seen, aging can have a variety of effects on your body. When it comes to metabolism, it shows that aging doesn't only affect your muscles, bones, and blood vessels; it can also affect the smallest cells in your body. As we grow older, our metabolism tends to slow down. It's almost like an engine that loses a bit of its horsepower. There is one drastic side effect of a declining metabolism—unwanted weight gain (uugh) and decreased energy levels (blaah).

To look at this closely, you will need to understand the scientific part, where metabolism is the chemical process that occurs in your body to maintain your life and energy production (*Metabolism: What It Is, How It Works and Disorders,* n.d.). It involves two components: Your body needs a specific number of calories to perform basic functions at rest, which include breathing, circulating blood, and maintaining your body temperature. This is usually around 60% to 70% of your daily energy expenditure. In addition, there is also the energy required to digest and absorb food, as well as contribute to your overall daily energy expenditure by moving, thinking, and so forth. When your metabolism decreases, your body will require fewer calories to perform its basic functions. This means that even if you eat the same amount of food, more will be stored as surplus, or fat, and this will lead to weight gain, as your body isn't using as much energy as before. There will also be reduced physical activity levels, as you feel lethargic and less motivated to engage in physical activities due to lower energy levels. With a sluggish metabolism, your appetite is also altered, making it more challenging to control food intake and resulting in overeating.

Strategies for an Efficient Metabolism

To avoid the side effects of aging on your metabolism, you will need to fuel it. This starts with what is on your plate and extends to your lifestyle habits. Let's look at the strategies that you could implement to boost your metabolism.

The first step is to include lean proteins in your diet. This includes chicken, fish, beans, and tofu. These foods require more energy to digest, which gives your metabolism a boost. Avoid eating foods that are rich in sugar, as this will only result in early digestion and absorption, which require very little energy usage. The disadvantage of eating foods containing sugar is that the sugar is converted into energy and is stored. Try to eat foods that do not get converted into fat. If you are interested in finding out what types of carbohydrates to add to your diet, always rely on complex carbohydrates, which take some time before getting digested.

The second step is to begin strength-training exercises. The reason why this type of exercise is more beneficial when it comes to your metabolism is one that we have already looked at. With strength training, you are specifically targeting your muscles and your strength. This means that as you continue with these exercises, you are going to become stronger, which results in growing muscles. This growth in muscles will cause a reversal in what has been happening in your body due to aging. Remember that muscles tend to use up energy even while they are at rest. This means that the more muscular you are, the more energy your body will use while you are at rest, and even more energy is used when you are active.

This is another great way to achieve weight reduction or at least manage it.

The next step is to constantly hydrate. With dehydration, your metabolism slows down. If you can't drink a lot of water in one go, try to sip water throughout the day to keep your engine running smoothly. Remember, water is another very important aspect of your body. In fact, more than 70% of your body is made up of water, and without it, several processes and functions will stall. For this reason, it's important that you continuously keep your body hydrated, as there is more than just one benefit that comes from this.

Of every habit that we should incorporate, another crucial one is adequate sleep. Sometimes, we tend to imagine that sleeping for longer periods means that we are lazy. However, this is untrue, as the whole body needs sleep, and not just to feel rejuvenated the next day. Without adequate sleep, hormones are disrupted, affecting appetite and metabolism. In fact, other processes are also hindered or affected in some major way. You should always aim for seven to nine hours of quality sleep each night to ensure that your body is working and functioning as it should. By depriving your body of sleep, you are pulling the plug on an efficient and healthy action, both physical and mental , for your well-being.

You should also try to spice it up when it comes to your meals. There are certain spices, like chili peppers, that contain compounds that temporarily increase your metabolism. Sometimes a bland diet means a dull life. You should try to add some spices, as foods are known to have some superpowers in them as well. Try out some spices that are known for their medicinal properties. Turmeric, Ginger, Cumin, Echinacea, and others.

The next step is to ensure that you are eating regular meals. As you skip meals, your metabolism goes into hibernation mode. This means that your body feels as though it is going through a starvation phase. Whatever you eat will then be saved or stored as fat for later use. However, with regular meals, your body knows that it is going to be getting food regularly and it does not need to store it for later, but it can use the necessary amount of energy it needs throughout the day.

As you incorporate these strategies into your daily life, your metabolism will be boosted, and you will notice how much more of a positive effect it has on your mood and overall well-being.

THE GUT MICROBIOME

Recently, new information about the gut microbiome has been taking up the headlines. In the intricate landscape of nutrition and health, there is a bustling city you might not have even been aware of, and this is your microbiome. Over the years, research has gone into the digestive system to find out just what exactly occurs there. From this research, it was found that there is a thriving community of trillions of microorganisms that cause the gastrointestinal tract to call home. However, the microbiome doesn't only exist here; it exists on your skin, as well as other mucosal membranes. The reason why the microbiome came as a shock to the medical community is because of just how important it is to your daily lifestyle and activities (*National Institute of Environmental Health Sciences*, 2022).

The Gut Microbiome Unveiled

One would imagine that if there is such an ecosystem of trillions of microorganisms living within the gut, its sole purpose is digestion. However, this is not true. This ecosystem of microorganisms plays a pivotal role in digestion, immune function, and mood regulation. It even goes on to regulate and secrete certain hormones that are necessary for your body's daily processes.

The Relationship With Nutrition

- Another misconception that many people tend to believe is that whatever we eat is okay for the gut microbiome. This is also very untrue. The foods you eat are very important, not just for your own body but for the microbiome as well. As is true for your body, different foods have different values, and some foods are detrimental to your gut

> instead of beneficial. It is a similar situation for your microbiome. Certain foods have a positive effect, while others have a negative one. And there are specific foods, known as prebiotics, that nourish specific types of bacteria in your digestive system. These foods are so important that they actually shape the composition of the microbial community in your gut.

Examples of prebiotics include:

- inulin, a type of prebiotic fiber that is found in various plant foods; natural sources include Jerusalem artichokes, garlic, and chicory root
- many fruits and vegetables like bananas, onions, leeks, and asparagus
- some legumes and certain dairy products, for example, beans, lentils, and chickpeas
- seaweed
- whole grains
- green, leafy vegetables
- fruits with their skin

If you incorporate foods that are rich in prebiotic fibers that will feed the microbes in your microbiome, you will benefit more than one area of your body.

Now you will ask, "What exactly influences the microbiome other than food? What should I avoid?"

It is quite obvious that your dietary choices will have a profound impact on your gut microbiome.

- Always try to incorporate a diet rich in fiber from fruits, vegetables, and whole grains to promote the growth of beneficial bacteria in your body.
- Try to avoid excessive sugar and processed foods, which directly lead to an overgrowth of harmful microbes in your body.
- Keep in mind that processed foods have no beneficial properties and, instead, inflame your gut lining.
- Processed foods also have an abundance of harmful microbes within them.
- Another addition to your diet would be probiotics and fermented foods. These two are great at introducing beneficial bacteria into your gut. Try to eat fermented foods like yogurt, kimchi, and kefir, which are all-natural sources of probiotics that will help maintain a healthy balance in your microbiome.
- One issue that many people overlook is the impact of antibiotics on your gut microbiome. Antibiotics are specifically designed to kill bacteria. However, the only issue is that they are unable to differentiate between good and bad bacteria. When you take antibiotics to treat infections, they can inadvertently disrupt your gut microbiome. For this reason, whenever you are prescribed

antibiotics, you should follow your healthcare provider's instructions carefully and consider taking probiotic supplements to support your gut health.

- Another point to consider is stress management. With heightened emotions, your stress levels can increase, which can affect the composition of your gut microbiome. By incorporating certain practices, like mindfulness and relaxation techniques, you can help maintain a healthy balance.
- Avoid overusing disinfectants and anti-bacterial products, as these can alter the microbial ecosystem in your environment and potentially affect your gut microbiome as well.
- Drink enough water to maintain a healthy gut lining, which supports a balanced microbiome.

As you make mindful choices about your diet and lifestyle, you can foster a flourishing gut microbiome, which contributes to your overall health and vitality.

THE USDA RECOMMENDED DAILY NUTRITION

Let's take a brief look at what the U.S. Department of Agriculture stipulates as guidelines for daily nutrition to promote your health and well-being (USDA, 2020).

- From the list of macronutrients, carbohydrates should make up about 40% to 70% of your daily calorie intake. Always try to choose complex carbohydrates like whole grains, fruits, and vegetables over simple sugars. The reason why these complex carbs are important is because they are broken down in the gut and used for energy to sustain your life and ensure that you are capable of fulfilling day-to-day tasks. Complex carbs also act as a source of food for your gut microbiome.
- The next nutrient is protein. This nutrient should account for about 10% to 40% of your daily calories. Some of the sources include poultry, fish, beans, and tofu. Always remember that you can obtain protein even from foods that are not in the meat category. You can get protein from lentils as well as dairy alternatives. If you aren't comfortable with any of these choices, you could always get your daily protein intake from food supplements.
- The next nutrient on your list is healthy fats, which should contribute to about 20% to 40% of your daily calories. You should focus on unsaturated fats like those found in fish, seeds, nuts, and avocados. As you incorporate these healthy fats into your diet, try to eliminate saturated and trans fats from your daily meals. This includes margarine or butter, some commercially baked foods, and some

hydrogenated oils. Saturated fats are found in animal products like full-fat dairy products, fatty cuts of meat, poultry with skin, and whole milk. You could also find it in coconut oil, processed foods, and some tropical oils like palm or cocoa butter.

Now we come to our list of micronutrients, which includes vitamins.

- Always try to consume a variety of fruits and vegetables to ensure that you're getting a wide range of vitamins, which include vitamins A, D, C, and B.
- From this, there are minerals, which include calcium, which can be found in dairy products and fortified plant-based alternatives; potassium, which can be found in bananas, potatoes, and leafy green vegetables; and iron, which can be found in lean meats, beans, and fortified cereals.
- You should also try to incorporate at least 25 grams of fiber per day for women and 38 grams for men. You could find fiber in whole grains, legumes, fruits, and vegetables.
- Sodium, on the other hand, should be limited to less than a teaspoon per day. By reducing the amount of sodium in your diet, you can reduce the risk of developing hypertension.

- We now come to added sugars, which should be less than 10% of your daily calories. They are usually found in sugary beverages, chocolates, and sweets.

Now you have a valuable road map to help you make informed decisions and choices about your daily nutrition so as to support your health and well-being. Let's move to the Mediterranean diet and what makes it so exceptional in nurturing both your gut and your well-being.

THE MEDITERRANEAN DIET

When we speak of the Mediterranean diet, it's more than just food; it's a lifestyle that is celebrated for its important role in promoting health and longevity. At its core, it's mainly a plant-based diet that is inspired by the traditional eating patterns of countries that border the Mediterranean Sea. Let's explore this diet in more detail (Gunnars, 2021).

These recipes usually emphasize certain ingredients, which include plenty of fruits and vegetables, nuts, legumes, and whole grains.

You may wonder why these types of meals are considered the healthiest dietary options. These foods are rich in calcium from dietary products and fortified plant-based alternatives. They are also rich in bone-building nutrients like vitamin D and magnesium from foods that include leafy green vegetables and fish. When you put all of these elements together, they support bone health while reducing the risk of mineral bone density reduction, as well as fractures as you age.

Another great benefit of these foods is the heart-healthy fats they are famous for. With an emphasis on olive oil, nuts, and fatty fish like salmon, the foods are packed with omega-3 fatty acids and monounsaturated fats. They are essential when it comes to reducing bad cholesterol levels, lowering your blood pressure, and decreasing the risk of developing cardiovascular diseases. This is an important benefit that one could receive from meals alone, especially as you age. The great part about these meals and the cardiovascular benefits is that you don't have to work too hard with your workout routines to obtain them. Adding moderate exercise while enjoying healthy Mediterranean-style dishes will ensure that your heart is pumping for a long time.

Since the diet emphasizes fresh fruits, vegetables, and whole grains, it provides you with a wealth of antioxidants and nutrients that support your vascular health. This is very important when it comes to maintaining sexual capacity at your age. Then again, with a healthy cardiovascular system, there will be better blood flow, which contributes to overall sexual well-being. Your body is much more physically able.

With the abundance of antioxidants and anti-inflammatory foods from vegetables, fruits, and whole grains, there is another benefit your body receives: preserving cognitive function. This reduces the risk of cognitive decline, as well as neurodegenerative diseases, which include Alzheimer's and Parkinson's. With the right type of food, you can stay mentally sharp as you age. The mental benefits are numerous.

Since this is a diverse, plant-based diet with plenty of vitamins and minerals, it also helps boost your immune system. Protective foods are the main resource your body has for improving its immune system. Only with the right vitamins and minerals will it be able to target and fight off specific diseases and infections. Other than this, your immune system will also be able to prevent certain conditions from developing. There are various foods that are considered superfoods, and these are all-natural products. These foods contain specific vitamins and minerals, which all have specific purposes in the body. For example, vitamin A is beneficial when it comes to your eyesight, and vitamin D is beneficial when it comes to your bones. Vitamin C is very important when it comes to fighting off infections like the flu and colds.

Every one of nature's products out there has some kind of unique property that makes it beneficial to your body. A Mediterranean diet takes advantage of the fact that fruits and vegetables can become your medicine. For this reason, the essential nutrients you obtain from your diet help reduce the risk of dysregulation and susceptibility to infections.

Another great benefit of a Mediterranean diet is that there is a reduction in inflammation. As we have already seen, chronic inflammation is a driver of many age-related diseases and conditions. Since this diet focuses on anti-inflammatory foods such as nuts, colorful fruits and vegetables, spices, and fatty fish, it can all come together to help with inflammation, as well as potentially delay the onset of age-related health issues.

Basically, the Mediterranean diet is a treasure trove of health benefits that can help you on your journey to healthy aging. The emphasis on whole, nutrient-dense foods will help provide you with a holistic approach to maintaining your physical, emotional, and mental well-being. The great part about this is that you get to savor the flavors of the Mediterranean and toast to a vibrant, healthy future.

Now, to put the knowledge into action, let's take a look at some simple recipes that you could incorporate into your daily diet. These recipes are simple to make and consist of various nutrient-dense foods. If there are certain ingredients that you are unable to obtain, you could always replace them with a certain food group that is available to you. Remember to keep it light and fun, and you can always experiment to see what suits your taste and what doesn't.

SIMPLE AND EASY RECIPES

Mediterranean Breakfast Ideas

Greek Yogurt Parfait

Layer Greek yogurt with honey, fresh berries, and a sprinkle of granola for a delicious and nutritious start to your day.

Mediterranean Omelet

Whip up an omelet filled with spinach, tomatoes, feta cheese, a dash of oregano, and some salt and pepper to taste.

Avocado Toast

Top whole-grain toast with mashed avocado, cherry tomatoes, a drizzle of olive oil, and a pinch of sea salt.

Mediterranean Scrambled Eggs

Scramble eggs with diced red peppers, onions, a touch of feta cheese, and salt and pepper to taste.

Mediterranean Lunch Ideas

Greek Salad

Combine cucumbers, tomatoes, red onions, Kalamata olives, and feta cheese. Drizzle with olive oil and sprinkle with oregano.

Hummus and Veggie Wrap

Spread hummus on a whole-grain tortilla; add sliced cucumbers, red bell peppers, and baby spinach; and roll it up.

Mediterranean Quinoa Salad

Toss cooked quinoa with diced cucumbers, cherry tomatoes, red onion, parsley, and a lemon vinaigrette.

Mediterranean Dinner Ideas

Grilled Salmon

Season salmon with herbs and grill it. Serve with a side of steamed broccoli and quinoa.

Mediterranean Stuffed Peppers

Fill bell peppers with a mixture of ground turkey, brown rice, diced tomatoes, and Mediterranean spices. Bake until tender.

Chicken Souvlaki

Marinate chicken in lemon, garlic, and oregano, then grill or roast it. Serve with pita bread and tzatziki sauce.

Mediterranean Snack Ideas

Greek Tzatziki Dip

Pair cucumber and yogurt-based tzatziki with whole-grain pita bread or carrot sticks for dipping.

Olives and Nuts

Mix a handful of olives and unsalted nuts for a satisfying and heart-healthy snack.

Hummus and Veggies

Dip baby carrots, cherry tomatoes, and cucumber slices into creamy hummus.

Mediterranean Dessert Ideas

Fruit Salad

Combine fresh seasonal fruits like oranges, grapes, and pomegranate seeds. Drizzle with honey and sprinkle with chopped mint leaves.

Baklava

This is regarded as an indulgent dessert; a small piece of this sweet, nut-filled pastry can be a delightful treat on occasion.

Now that you have some recipes to play around with, let's look at a specifically tailored diet plan for you that comes with a few meal ideas you can incorporate into your daily diet. You can choose to follow this plan or mix it up a little to suit your preferences. Remember to keep it natural and Mediterranean.

A Mediterranean Meal Plan

Day 1

- Breakfast: Greek yogurt parfait
- Lunch: Greek salad
- Dinner: grilled salmon with quinoa and broccoli
- Snack: hummus and veggie sticks

Day 2

- Breakfast: Mediterranean omelet
- Lunch: hummus and veggie wrap
- Dinner: Mediterranean stuffed peppers
- Snack: olives and nuts

Day 3

- Breakfast: avocado spread on two slices of brown toast
- Lunch: Mediterranean quinoa salad topped with nuts of your choice
- Dinner: chicken souvlaki with tzatziki
- Snack: Fruit salad

Days 4 to 7

Repeat the above meal plan or mix and match your favorite Mediterranean breakfast, lunch, and dinner ideas. Incorporate your favorite fruits, veggies, and whole grains into the mix. Experiment and even come up with your own fun ideas. I have tried to keep this section brief, one quick internet search for Mediterranean Diet will give you countless hours of meal ideas.

As we come to the end of this chapter, remember that even though physical health is paramount, your emotional well-being and social interaction are equally crucial for aging well. In the next chapter, we're going to explore the intricate connection between your emotional health and overall well-being as we dive deep into strategies that will help you maintain your mental and emotional vitality on your journey through life.

6

ENHANCING EMOTIONAL HEALTH AND SOCIAL INTERACTION

> *The greatest health is wealth.*
>
> — VIRGIL

When we think of the grand symphony of life, we realize that health is the most coveted treasure. Without it, we are nothing; and without it, there is no future. Without it, there is no need to plan and see our goals achieved. With an unhealthy lifestyle, there is only deterioration, pain, and negativity. We have spiraled downward from what life is truly meant to be.

Then again, health isn't only about our physical aspects. It isn't about our muscles or bones, how strong we are, or how capable we are of lifting and pushing things. Health also encompasses our emotional well-being and the invaluable tapestry of social interactions. This we can glean from the words of Virgil.

In the last chapter of this book, we are going to embark on a journey that explores the intricate world of how emotional health, as well as significant social interactions, provides us with life. So, what is the goal? We are going to equip you with strategies to counter stress, find inner peace, and cultivate all of those rich, meaningful social connections that enrich our lives.

EMOTIONAL HEALTH AND WELL-BEING

Try to picture your emotions and feelings as vibrant flowers growing in a garden. Your emotional health should be an internal garden that you tend to frequently. Most of the time, we overlook our emotions and mental health. We tend to focus only on our physical body and what we are experiencing in our muscles, joints, and bones. However, as we have already mentioned, our body is made up of more than just our physical aspects. Our emotional health matters more than we think.

Another misconception that we tend to believe is that our emotional aspect is only about feeling happiness and avoiding negativity. This is not true; in fact, our emotional health is more about the ability to navigate all of life's ups and downs, challenges, and opportunities with resilience and grace. Think of it as a sturdy boat that helps you sail through stormy seas, emerging stronger on the other side.

Your physical body is full of externals, while your emotional side is more about who you are within. Then again, with healthy aging, you can't just worry about what your body is experiencing. You also must think about what your mind is going through. Aging doesn't only take a toll on your physical aspects but on your mental capabilities and form as well.

As we age, we don't only feel it in our body mechanics. We also feel it in our minds. We feel our mental health degrading; we feel our memory becoming more affected; and we feel our mental strength draining. We also feel that the sort of negative impact bouncing off the mental shield we try to install day in and day out. The bottom line is that our emotional health isn't just a warm and fuzzy concept; it's tightly intertwined with our overall well-being. It's like the conductor of a band who is leading the way the music flows, orchestrating it from a harmonious relationship between your mind and body and then making you notice it as a singular aspect when the music stops and all you can hear is the singer's voice. Most of the time, we do not notice the value of our emotional health, but it is the one thing that helps us get out of every tricky situation we get into, especially when it comes to the side effects of aging.

Let's move on to the next part of this emotional journey, where you learn how to unravel the mysteries of your emotions and equip yourself with powerful tools to manage them.

RESPOND, DON'T REACT

When it comes to the grand theater of life, emotional regulation takes center stage. Basically, it's all about encouraging thoughtful responses rather than being a puppet of knee jerk reactions.

If we think of it, there's always one person in our lives who remains remarkably composed, even when facing catastrophe. We always wish that we could develop the same kind of reaction or response system that they have. Then again, no matter how much we try or think we are trying, we can never do it right. How are these people mastering the art of responding rather than reacting?

To answer this, it all boils down to emotional regulation. This is where you must try to imagine that your emotions are waves in the ocean. Reacting is as though you are being tossed around by those waves, and the toll is only waiting for you to take some kind of impulsive action or say some words that you will later regret. Responding on the other side is similar to navigating the rocky waves and ensuring that you stay on course. You aren't affected by what is going on around you, as you can think clearly and navigate the right route.

This concept of emotional regulation isn't about suppressing your emotions. You do feel the normal flare of emotions, except that you understand how to manage them. There are a few techniques that you can incorporate to help you become the captain of your emotional ship as you decide and steer where you want to go.

First, we have deep-breathing exercises where you get to feel the emotional tension, and then you learn to take a moment to breathe deeply. You inhale serenity and exhale the stress. It's a very simple act that can help calm down your nervous system and provide your mind with some clarity. To do this, whenever you are facing a difficult situation, instead of reacting, close your eyes as soon as you notice that the situation is going downhill. Instead of opening your mouth to speak, take a deep breath in and hold it in your chest as you feel your reactions letting go. As you breathe out, you expel the tension and let go. Repeat this process for a few seconds until you feel that you are capable of responding to the situation with calm and clarity.

Second, you will need to take a step back. It's important that you learn to train yourself so that whenever a situation becomes heated, your mind and judgment aren't clouded. As soon as you feel your temper or emotions rising, take a step back to calm yourself. You can envision yourself stepping off the hotplate and cooling down, reviewing the situation, and then making a decision about what to say or which path to take.

Third, you need to encourage a stronger inner dialogue. This is what eventually helps shape your emotional responses and replaces the negative self-talk with positive ones. You become capable of changing the way your mind thinks by silently speaking to yourself, feeding your thoughts more positivity rather than allowing negativity to rule. Replace negative self-talk with positive affirmations. Instead of saying, "I can't handle this," say, "I am capable, and I'll tackle this step by step, one piece at a time."

Take time to teach yourself to look at things more deeply than they seem. Find the cause of the situation. See how you can solve the problem instead of just defending yourself and what you've done. Try to look for the problem and what your part is, as well as how you can solve it. This will make you look at situations differently. Instead of immediately jumping to negative thoughts or feelings in a heated situation, you should stop and look at the other side. How do you deal with an issue? By solving it and not just standing up for yourself or backing yourself up, you become capable of looking at the situation as a whole. We often see things in only one direction. But by developing this kind of mindset, situations are quickly diffused, and emotions can be regulated without too much effort.

Now that we have some insight on how to deal with fluctuating emotions, let's move on to stress.

Strategies for Stress Reduction

Stress is a natural part of life. We have already gone over this aspect in an earlier chapter, but now it's time to look into it deeply. We know that chronic stress can wreak havoc on not just our mental health but our physical health as well. It's detrimental, and it wouldn't be far-fetched to assume that more than half of the population suffers from it, but they feel that there's nothing much to do about it, so it's ignored. However, this is not the correct mentality to have when dealing with stress. To put it mildly, yes, stress is a universal adversary, but you don't have to be its perpetual victim. Let's arm you with strategies to not just cope with stress but conquer it.

- You can engage in physical activity, as this isn't just physical fitness but also a formidable way to tackle stress. We have looked at this previously, but engaging in regular physical activity will help release endorphins into your bloodstream. These are natural mood-enhancing chemicals that help you de-stress and become a much more positive and happy individual. If you haven't started with physical activity before, now that you have a great source of motivation, you want to cut down on that stress. Start off small, like taking a daily walk, and gradually build up from there to more rigorous activities like jogging, running, and other types of exercise.
- You can also start cultivating a hobby. With hobbies as creative or interactive outlets, it creates a bubble around you where stress struggles to find a foothold. It doesn't matter what kind of hobby it

is—painting, gardening, learning to play an instrument, or even immersing yourself in a book —this provides a welcome escape from daily pressures. With hobbies, you get to find some sense of purpose and fulfillment.

- Another strategy that you could incorporate is utilizing relaxation techniques. There are quite a few that you could try to see which one suits you best. In the end, they all work toward one goal—decreasing stress levels and enhancing, as well as improving, your relaxation levels. As you learn from these techniques and incorporate them into your daily routines, you will learn how to control your stress levels. Let's look at some of the different relaxation techniques that you can use.

Deep Breathing

This is a common relaxation technique that is simple to do. You should:

- Find a quiet and comfortable place to sit or lie down.
- Close your eyes as you begin to take a deep breath through your nose.
- Hold your breath for a few seconds before exhaling slowly and completely through your mouth.

- The duration of your inhale and exhale should not be less than four seconds.
- Repeat this breathing pattern several times as you focus on your breath and let go of the tension with every exhale.

Progressive Muscle Relaxation

This involves tensing and relaxing your muscles. To do this, you should:

- Start with the movements of your toes as you work your way up, or you can start from the top and then move to the bottom.
- You should tense each muscle group in your body for about 5 to 10 seconds and then relax that muscle group for 20 to 30 seconds.
- Pay attention to the sensations of tension and relaxation as you move through each muscle.
- Continue this movement until you've relaxed all the major muscle groups in your body.

Visualization

This is where you use your imagination and your mind to help calm and relax your emotions and stress levels. To do this, you should:

- Find a calm and quiet place to practice.
- Begin by sitting down and then closing your eyes as you begin to imagine a peaceful and tranquil place. Some examples include a beach, a forest, or a natural oasis you always thought of as peaceful.
- Begin to pick up on the sights, sounds, and sensations as much as you can. Try to look at every detail.
- Move toward engaging your senses in this mental journey as you focus on being present in that visualization.
- You should be relaxed and tranquil.

Guided Imagery

This is an activity where you use guided imagery audio recordings or even a smartphone app to help you along this path. You will need to follow the narrator's instructions as the individual leads you through a relaxing mental journey. This technique helps you visualize and experience a sense of calm and peace without having to do anything except listen to their voice as it guides you.

Other techniques include:

- Aromatherapy is where you choose a calming essential oil like lavender, eucalyptus, or chamomile and use an essential oil diffuser. Another way to make use of the oils is by adding a few drops to a bowl of warm water. You inhale the soothing aroma, which allows you to relax your mind and body.

- Yoga and stretching are practices where you pay attention to your breath and the sensations of your body as you move through each pose or stretch. These tend to help relieve physical tension while promoting relaxation.
- Tai chi and Chi Gong.
- Go for a nature walk or try progressive relaxation apps like Calm, Headspace, or Insight Timer.

Remember that different relaxation techniques work differently for each person, and it's essential that you find the one that resonates with you. These strategies aren't just emergency tools; you should remember to use them daily to help build resilience, nurture emotional health, and create a foundation for more meaningful social interactions.

THE POWER OF GRATITUDE

When it comes to aspects of emotional health, gratitude is a vibrant thread that adds depth, color, and resilience to emotions. It's not just a polite gesture; it's more of a pulling force that can transform your life. This is similar to optimism, as we have looked at previously. It's not just one feeling or way of looking at life. With gratitude, there is more than one way of defining it. It is the art of recognizing and appreciating the good in your life, no matter how small or unimportant certain things may be. Most wise men over the years have always said that we should be grateful. We should look at our lives, and even though all we see is a battlefield, we should still be appreciative of the little things that we have had over the years.

What does this mean? By appreciating every good and bad thing you have come across, you receive the antidote to the poison of negativity and stress. How does all of this relate to emotional health? When you practice gratitude—which is going back and being appreciative of everything you have experienced, gained, and lost over the years—you are rewiring your brain to focus only on the positive. Even if there was negativity, you are grateful for what the negative moments taught you and what they took away that might have been an issue down the line. You get to celebrate what you have now instead of focusing on what is missing. Shifting your perspective can have a profound impact on your emotional well-being.

Aging comes with its own set of challenges, from physical ailments to changing social dynamics. We have looked at more than a few side effects of growing older, but there is a secret weapon that can change the entire journey. This is gratitude. As you embrace gratitude and incorporate it as a way of life, it can help you navigate the challenges of aging with resilience and grace. Courage is a sense of fulfillment and contentment that counters negative feelings of loneliness or isolation. It also tends to foster optimism, which is an elixir of youth that keeps your spirit young and vibrant. Remember, your physical body is not your whole self. Your emotional side makes up half of you. By getting your emotional well-being in tip-top shape, you will be able to live a more vibrant and fulfilling life.

The Gratitude Journal

Now that you understand the benefits of embracing gratitude and incorporating it into your daily outlook on life, you will ask the question, "How do I harness the magic of gratitude when it didn't come naturally before?

The most powerful way is to use a gratitude journal. This is a very simple practice that involves writing down the things you are grateful for each day. It's almost like collecting treasures of joy and appreciating them. You get to write them down so you can always visit them whenever you feel as though negativity might be taking control again.

Beginning this gratitude journal can be quite a challenge, as staring at a blank page can be intimidating. However, don't worry, as we have got you covered with over 50 prompts to help kick-start your gratitude journey. Let's discover them now.

- Write about the one thing you are thankful for in your morning routine.
- Write about a cherished memory from your childhood that is still vivid in your mind. Write

about why you cherish it, as well as how it makes you feel.

- Reflect on a past friendship or relationship that brought you joy. Write about the person and why you still remember them.
- Reflect on a moment when you felt truly content and at peace with yourself.
- Write about a valuable life lesson you've learned from a difficult experience.
- Express gratitude for the simple pleasures of everyday life, like a warm cup of tea or a cozy blanket.
- Think about a time when you felt a strong sense of belonging or connection with others.
- Write about a skill or hobby you've developed over time that brings you joy.
- Reflect on a favorite piece of clothing or accessory and the memories associated with it.
- Express thanks for the freedom and independence you've enjoyed throughout your life.
- Think about a place you've lived in the past and what you appreciated about it.
- Write about a charitable or community event you've been a part of and the positive impact it had.
- Reflect on the beauty of the night sky or a particularly memorable sunrise or sunset.
- Express gratitude for the beauty of nature. What do you love about the outdoors?

- Think about a specific skill or talent you possess and how it has enriched your life.
- Write a note of appreciation to someone who has made a positive impact on your life.
- What is your favorite book, movie, or piece of music that has brought you happiness?
- Describe a recent experience that made you laugh or smile.
- Recall a meal or dish that you particularly enjoyed and express gratitude for it.
- Reflect on a moment when you felt proud of an accomplishment.
- What aspects of your health and well-being are you grateful for today?
- Write about a place you've visited that holds special meaning for you.
- Express thanks for the support of family members, friends, or caregivers in your life.
- Think about a personal quality or characteristic that you value in yourself.
- Recall a time when you overcame a challenge or adversity and express gratitude for your resilience.
- Reflect on a historical event or time period that you find interesting or significant.
- Write about a simple pleasure or comfort in your daily life.
- What is a piece of advice or wisdom that has guided you through life?

- Express gratitude for the opportunity to learn and grow, no matter your age.
- Write about your hopes and dreams for the future and express thanks for the possibilities that lie ahead.
- Think about a time when someone showed you kindness. How did it make you feel?
- Reflect on a favorite holiday or celebration and what you appreciate most about it.
- Write about a piece of art—whether it's a painting, sculpture, or piece of music—that you find inspiring.
- Express gratitude for the modern conveniences and technologies that make life easier.
- Recall a teacher, mentor, or coach who had a positive influence on your life.
- Write about a time when you were able to help or support someone in need.
- Reflect on the changing seasons and what you enjoy about each one.
- Express your thanks for the wisdom and life lessons you've gained over the years.
- Think about a beloved pet or animal that has brought joy into your life.
- Write about a friendship that has endured through the years and why it's meaningful to you.
- Express gratitude for your senses (sight, hearing, taste, touch, and smell) and the experiences they bring.

- Recall a time when you were in a beautiful or tranquil natural setting.
- Write about a tradition or ritual that holds significance in your life.
- Reflect on a historical figure or role model who has inspired you.
- Express thanks for the opportunities you've had to travel and explore new places.
- Think about a positive change you've made in your life and how it has benefited you.
- Write about a specific hobby or interest that brings you joy and fulfillment.
- Express gratitude for the ability to reminisce and share stories with loved ones.
- Reflect on a cultural or religious practice that brings meaning to your life.
- Write about the love and affection you have for your family and specific moments that have strengthened those bonds.

Always remember to choose from those that resonate with you most.

Apart from journaling you could also:

- Start every day with a gratitude mantra or affirmation.
- Express your appreciation verbally to friends and loved ones.

- Keep a gratitude jar where you add notes of thanks when something good happens. You can pay it forward by performing random acts of kindness and using downtime to meditate on the things that you are grateful for.

By making gratitude a habit, you will enhance your emotional well-being.

FINDING PEACE IN DAILY LIFE

Amid the hustle and bustle of our daily lives, the pursuit of peace can feel as though it is a non-existent and fleeting dream. However, it is a state of being that you can nurture, not something that you have to look far and wide for. A fun fact is that for most if not all, tranquility lies in the embrace of nature. You should step outside, breathe in the fresh air, and let the symphony of the birds and rustling leaves soothe your soul.

Where to Look

Nature

Our surroundings offer a respite from the digital chaos that surrounds us. Nature is a reminder of the world's timeless beauty.

Being Present

Another avenue to finding your inner self is mindfulness. This is the state of being fully present in the moment. With this state of mind, you get to savor every experience, no matter how small or large. To do this, you need to practice mindfulness in every task and waking moment. Drink your morning coffee with intention as you feel the warmth of the sun on your skin with every sunrise. Relish the taste of a favorite meal instead of just swallowing it down while focusing on the TV. These simple acts can transform your boring and mundane moments into ones of profound peace and enjoyment.

Meditation and Spirituality

This is another powerhouse that leads to peace and tranquility—an elixir of emotional health. It is an inward journey, a pathway to obtaining stillness amidst the storms of life.

The benefits of meditation include

- stress-reduction
- refreshing your mind and spirit
- rewiring your mind to stop racing thoughts

There are different types of meditation, all of which have their own unique purpose. Whether it's mindfulness meditation for being present and in the moment, loving-kindness meditation that builds compassion, or transcendental meditation for deep relaxation, there is a technique for everyone and every circumstance. Let's look at a few practices you could try with some simple meditation tips.

Mindful Breathing

The steps:

- Focus on your breath as you inhale and exhale slowly.
- When your mind or your thoughts begin to wander, gently guide your focus back to your breath.
- Continue breathing in and out gently as you keep your mind calm and focused.

Body Scan

The steps:

- Begin by mentally scanning your body from head to toe.
- As you focus on each part, try to visualize yourself releasing tension from that body part as you continue moving forward.
- Try to cover every muscle group, organ, and bone.

Guided Meditation

Listen to a guided meditation recording that allows someone else to help guide you into a relaxed state with their soothing voice and relaxing commands. An easy way to find guided meditation videos is on YouTube.

SPIRITUALITY AND AGING

Spirituality is a guiding light throughout life. As we age, it becomes more important. It provides us with comfort, purpose, and a sense of connection to something greater than ourselves. Spirituality respects personal beliefs, and it is a deeply personal journey.

Building Social Connections

As we journey through life, there's one undeniable truth: Our social connections are like the secret glue that holds together our longevity.

With meaningful interactions and community involvement, there is some kind of magic that erupts that is a vital ingredient for aging well. A very fun way to discover why this magic or secret exists is written in our history, the Bible, and our mythology.

Man could not exist alone, so God created a woman to keep him company. The story of Adam and Eve is well known. However, from this, we learn one thing: No man is capable of living alone. It is true that in our current society, we value our privacy and quiet times. In fact, we do need some quiet time away from the noise, as this is very important when it comes to reducing our stress levels. However, by being together, socializing, and enjoying our time with others, this also acts as a stress reliever. From a mythical standpoint, man and woman were once one being. This can be found in Greek mythology, where long ago Zeus created people as beings stuck together. Eventually, the story went on to say that Zeus became scared of the power that people had when they were together and so he struck them down, cutting them into pieces. For this reason, men and women tend to seek companionship as they try to become stronger.

The funny thing is that with companionship, we are fulfilled. We have someone to talk to, share our experiences with, and create rivalries and bonds with. People share one similarity, and that is that we want to have other like-minded people in our lives. The main reason for this is that social connections are a part of who we are.

The Importance of Friends and Family

The bonds we share with our family and friends are like treasure chests that grow more valuable with time. With age, we realize that certain things aren't as important as we thought, and relationships with the people we love and care for are invaluable. They provide us with support, laughter, and a profound sense of belonging.

How to Build Strong Connections

To build stronger relationships:

- Always initiate contact; don't wait for others.
- Reach out regularly.
- Pursue hobbies or interests that bring you joy and connect you with other like-minded individuals.
- Volunteer and give back to your community, so as to make a positive impact.

Always remember that you don't have to wait for things to come to you. You have the ability to change your life. You have the power to make the things that you want and wish for in your life happen. All it takes is to make that first decision and take that step forward.

In conclusion, the tapestry of healthy aging is woven from numerous threads—physical health, emotional well-being, and social connections. The journey will have some challenges, but it's always worth it. Change can be daunting, but it is the vehicle that will transport you toward a healthier, happier, longer life. Don't wait. Embrace it, cherish it, and embark on this remarkable voyage toward a more vibrant, healthier, and better you.

KEEPING THE GAME ALIVE

Now you have everything you need to achieve a healthier, longer, stronger life. It's time to pass on your new found knowledge and show other readers where they can find the same help.

Simply by leaving your honest opinion of this book on Amazon, you'll show other Healthy Agers where they can find the information they're looking for, and pass their passion for Healthy Aging and Longevity forward.

Thank you for your help. Healthy Aging and Longevity is kept alive when we pass on our knowledge – and you're helping us to do just that.

Scan the QR code below to leave your review on Amazon

CONCLUSION: YIELDING TO CHANGE

As we near the end of our journey through these pages of *Discover Healthy Aging and Longevity,* I would like to leave with you a quote that encapsulates the message woven within every page: "The secret of change is to focus all of your energy not on fighting the old but on building the new". These words are by Dan Millman, who taught us that change is not about erasing past habits but, rather, about channeling your energy into building healthier and new ones.

Throughout this journey, we dug deep into the various aspects of aging: how we perceive it, observing our health, finding motivation, revitalizing our lives, nourishing our bodies, and supporting our emotional well-being. The message is clear: Healthy aging is not a myth or some far-fetched ideal. It is not a distant dream but an achievable reality that every one of us is capable of reaching.

In the first chapter, we challenged the stereotype that aging leads to a declining life. We looked through and acquired the wisdom and richness that each passing year can bring. Age is not an enemy but more of a valuable ally in the quest for a fulfilling life.

The second chapter guided you into looking closely at your health. You were encouraged to become a much more active participant in observing your health rather than watching it pass by slipping out of your hands. Your health will always be your most precious asset, and it is up to you to make decisions about what comes next. Do you need to make informed choices and protect what you have?

In the third chapter, the spark of motivation grows. You got to see the importance of setting goals, staying curious, and finding the purpose behind your life to keep you on the path toward achieving, obtaining, and helping others. You discovered this journey shouldn't only be about what you gain; it's also about what you eventually teach to others.

Chapter Four explored the power of revitalization through exercise as we age. We saw people who changed the direction of their lives, all with a little added activity here and there—something that became a fun and solid part of their everyday lives. We saw several types of exercise and what they had to offer, from the lowest fitness levels to how they could move up the ladder to achieve the health they are striving for.

The next chapter took a deep dive into the vital role nutrition plays in aging. You obtained knowledge and some fun tips on how you can turn medicine into your food and food into medicine. This way, your body is nourished and one step closer to longevity, and a vibrant lifestyle.

Lastly, we looked at the often-underestimated power of emotional health and resilience in social interaction. We looked at the significance of staying actively connected with others to foster emotional resilience and find joy in the little moments.

Now, as we reach the end, I'd like to share one last story to keep the seed of motivation growing. Emmy is a remarkable woman who, at the age of 66, decided to take up painting as a hobby. She had no prior experience but knew that she just wanted to do this. She embarked on this contemplative journey as she discovered a newfound passion that not only brought her immense joy but a sense of purpose as well. Through this hobby, she found a creative outlet. She found a way to express herself, connect with others, and embrace change with open arms. This story serves as a testament to the transformative power of embracing change and pursuing passions at any age. All is possible as long as you do it. Knowing that you want to do it and succeeding is all that matters. It's not about where you've been or what you've always been doing. Throw out the stereotypical mindset about the old dog who cannot learn new tricks and plunge in. You can never go wrong in the face of positivity and optimism.

Now is the time for me to encourage you. Take what you have learned from the pages of this book and put it into practice. Start now and at a small, manageable pace. Whether it's by getting into shape, choosing the right workouts, inspiring healthy eating, finding the right method to ensure healthy emotions, or reconnecting with those forgotten ties, you can do it. This is not a journey that's too late to start. Make the decision and do it!

You can do it!

Before the end, I would like to invite you to share your progress, experiences, and successes with others. By doing so, you will inspire and motivate many more to begin their own journey toward healthy aging. Your story can spark a positive change in someone else's life. Please leave a review of this book. Your feedback will not only help others find the transformative power in healthy aging but also motivate me to continue savoring the knowledge and inspiration I gain from wonderful readers like you.

Remember, the secret of change lies in your hands. Embrace every moment, relish every change, and build the life you've always dreamed of. This is your path toward healthy aging—a journey of self-discovery, growth, and fulfillment. Take hold of the path and never let go.

REFERENCES

Aging: What to expect. (2022, November 3). Mayo Clinic. https://www.mayoclinic.org/healthy-lifestyle/healthy-aging/in-depth/aging/art-20046070?reDate=14092023

A quote by William Shakespeare. (n.d.). Goodreads. https://www.goodreads.com/quotes/328938-our-bodies-are-our-gardens-to-which-our-wills-are

A quote by Virgil. (2019). Goodreads. https://www.goodreads.com/quotes/28440-the-greatest-wealth-is-health

Benefits of physical activity. (2021, November 1). Centers for Disease Control and Prevention. https://www.cdc.gov/physicalactivity/basics/pa-health/index.htm

Benefits of physical activity. (2022, April 27). Centers for Disease Control and Prevention. https://www.cdc.gov/physicalactivity/basics/pa-health/index.htm#:

Berger, R. (2017). Aging in America: Ageism and general attitudes toward growing old and the elderly. *Open Journal of Social Sciences, 05*(08), 183–198. https://doi.org/10.4236/jss.2017.58015

Biological and psychological aspects of aging. (n.d.). Wisconsin Technical College System. https://wtcs.pressbooks.pub/diversityintro/chapter/9-4-biological-and-psychological-aspects-of-aging

Cherry, K. (2023, May 3). *The psychology of what motivates us*. Verywell Mind. https://www.verywellmind.com/what-is-motivation-2795378#:

Day, D. (2022, June 14). *Activities and exercises to do outdoors*. Fourfive. https://fourfive.com/activities-and-exercises-to-do-outdoors

Dennis, H. (2021, December 5). *Why we fear aging and what we can do about it*. Daily News. https://www.dailynews.com/2021/12/05/why-we-fear-aging-and-what-we-can-do-about-it/amp

Dietary guidelines for Americans. (2020). USDA. https://www.dietaryguidelines.gov/sites/default/files/2020-12/Dietary_Guidelines_for_Americans_2020-2025.pdf

Elwood, P., Galante, J., Pickering, J., Palmer, S., Bayer, A., Ben-Shlomo, Y., Longley, M., & Gallacher, J. (2013). Healthy lifestyles reduce the incidence of chronic diseases and dementia: Evidence from the Caerphilly cohort study. *PLoS ONE, 8*(12), e81877. https://doi.org/10.1371/journal.pone.0081877

Ferrucci, L., & Fabbri, E. (2018). Inflammageing: chronic inflammation in ageing, cardiovascular disease, and frailty. *Nature Reviews Cardiology, 15*(9), 505–522. Research

Growing old in America: Expectations vs. reality. (2009, June 29). Pew Research Center. https://www.pewresearch.org/social-trends/2009/06/29/growing-old-in-america-expectations-vs-reality

Gunnars, K. (2021, October 25). *Mediterranean diet 101: Meal plan, foods list, and tips.* Healthline. https://www.healthline.com/nutrition/mediterranean-diet-meal-plan#what-is-it

Lane, E. (2021, March 11). *33 of the best beginner exercises to try at home for Burning Fat and Building Muscle.* Men's Health. https://www.menshealth.com/uk/building-muscle/a754099/the-15-best-beginners-exercises-to-do-at-home

Laskowski, E. R. (2023, July 26). *How much should the average adult exercise every day?* Mayo Clinic. https://www.mayoclinic.org/healthy-lifestyle/fitness/expert-answers/exercise/faq-20057916#:

Let food be thy medicine. (n.d.) Dr. Goodfood. https://www.drgoodfood.org/en/news/let-food-be-thy-medicine-hippocrates

Metabolism: What it is, how it works and disorders. (n.d.). Cleveland Clinic. https://my.clevelandclinic.org/health/body/21893-metabolism#:

Microbiome. (2022, April 5). National Institute of Environmental Health Sciences. https://www.niehs.nih.gov/health/topics/science/microbiome/index.cfm

Movement is a medicine for creating change in a person's physical, emotional, and mental states. (n.d.). Outdoor Mindset. https://www.outdoormindset.org/blog//2010/06/movement-is-medicine-for-creating.html#:

Schwartz, S. H. (2011). *An overview of the Schwartz theory of basic values.* ScholarWorks. https://scholarworks.gvsu.edu/orpc/vol2/iss1/11

Signs and symptoms of stress. (2022, March). Mind. https://www.mind.

org.uk/information-support/types-of-mental-health-problems/stress/signs-and-symptoms-of-stress

The 4 most important types of exercise. (2017, January 13). Harvard Health. https://www.health.harvard.edu/exercise-and-fitness/the-4-most-important-types-of-exercise

The microbiome. (2017, August 16). The Nutrition Source. https://www.hsph.harvard.edu/nutritionsource/microbiome/#:

What is mindfulness? (2020, July 8). Mindful. https://www.mindful.org/what-is-mindfulness/#:

You are never too old to set another goal or to dream a new dream. (2023, March 3). Medium. https://medium.com/@officialprpatel002/you-are-never-too-old-to-set-another-goal-or-to-dream-a-new-dream-c-s-lewis-e2e3d0e03d2f

Zhang, J.-M., & An, J. (2007). Cytokines, inflammation, and pain. *International Anesthesiology Clinics, 45*(2), 27–37.

Made in the USA
Columbia, SC
06 September 2024